PUBLIC HEALTH AND PREVENTIVE MEDICINE REVIEW

Second Edition

Rafael A. Peñalver, M.D.

Director, Office of International Medical Education
Clinical Professor of Occupational Medicine and Medicine
University of Miami School of Medicine
Miami, Florida
U.S.A.

**ARCO PUBLISHING, INC.
NEW YORK**

To
AURORITA
and to
RALPH, MANNY, ALBERTO, and AURORITICA

Second Edition, First Printing, 1984

Published by Arco Publishing, Inc.
215 Park Avenue South, New York, N.Y. 10003

Copyright © 1979, 1984 by Arco Publishing, Inc.

All rights reserved. No part of this book may be reproduced, by any means, without permission in writing from the publisher, except by a reviewer who wishes to quote brief excerpts in connection with a review in a magazine or newspaper.

Library of Congress Cataloging in Publication Data

Peñalver, Rafael A.
  Public health and preventive medicine review.

  (ARCO medical review series)
  Bibliography: p.
  1. Public health—Examinations, questions, etc.
2. Medicine, Preventive—Examinations, questions, etc.
I. Title. II. Series. [DNLM: 1. Preventive medicine.
2. Public health. WA 100 P397p]
RA430.P46 1984   614′.076   83-10033
ISBN 0-668-05936-2 (pbk.)

Printed in the United States of America

Contents

Preface — *iv*

References — *v*

Chapter 1	**Biostatistics and Population Dynamics**	1
	Answers and Explanations	17
Chapter 2	**Epidemiology**	29
	Answers and Explanations	45
Chapter 3	**Sexually Transmitted Diseases**	57
	Answers and Explanations	63
Chapter 4	**Nutrition and Deficiency Diseases**	67
	Answers and Explanations	71
Chapter 5	**Occupational Diseases of the Skin**	73
	Answers and Explanations	85
Chapter 6	**Occupational Lung Disorders**	93
	Answers and Explanations	96
Chapter 7	**Environmental Toxicology**	98
	Answers and Explanations	108
Chapter 8	**Effects of the Physical Environment**	115
	Answers and Explanations	119

Preface

The stimulus to write this book came from my participation as a faculty member in the programs for foreign medical graduates that are regularly offered at the University of Miami School of Medicine, Miami, Florida, and Saint Barnabas Medical Center, Livingston, New Jersey, U.S.A.; Rome University School of Medicine, Rome, Italy; Escuela de Medicina de la Universidad Autonoma de Guadalajara, Jalisco, Mexico; Escuela de Medicina de la Universidad Central del Este, San Pedro de Macoris, Dominican Republic; and Kuwait-Miami Comprehensive Medical Education Program, State of Kuwait — Arabian Gulf. More than 14,000 foreign medical graduates from more than 70 different countries have attended these courses.

This book consists of 1,000 questions and explained answers. The material is relevant for preparation for medical school examinations; for the Foreign Medical Graduate Examination in the Medical Sciences, administered by the Educational Commission for Foreign Medical Graduates (ECFMG); for the Federation Licensing Examination (FLEX); and for the American Board of Preventive Medicine examinations leading to certification in Public Health, Aerospace Medicine, Occupational Medicine, and General Preventive Medicine.

References

Below is a numbered list of reference works pertaining to the material in this book. On the last line of most explanations, at the right-hand side, there appears a number combination in parentheses that identifies the reference source and the page where the information relating to the question may be found. The first number refers to the work in the list, and the second number refers to the page of that work.

For example: (4:135) is a reference to the fourth book in the list, Barlow's *Sexually Transmitted Diseases,* page 135.

1. Adams RM: High-risk dermatoses. *Journal of Occupational Medicine* 23:829, 1981.
2. AMA Department of Drugs: *AMA Drug Evaluations.* American Medical Association, Chicago, 1980.
3. Barker DJP: *Practical Epidemiology.* Churchill Livingstone, Edinburgh, 1982.
4. Barlow D: *Sexually Transmitted Diseases.* Oxford University Press, Oxford, England, 1979.
5. Baselt RC: *Biological Monitoring Methods for Industrial Chemicals.* Biomedical Publications, Davis, Calif., 1980.
6. Benenson AS: *Control of Communicable Diseases in Man,* 13th ed. American Public Health Association, Washington, D.C., 1981.
7. Brewis RAL: *Lecture notes on Respiratory Disease.* Blackwell, Oxford, England, 1978.
8. Burton LLE, Smith HH, Nichols AW: *Public Health and Community Medicine,* 2nd ed. Williams & Wilkins, Baltimore, 1980.
9. CDC: *Health information for International Travel 1982.* MMWR Supplement. HHS Publication No. (CDC) 82-8280, Atlanta, 1982.
10. CDC: *Prevention of Malaria in Travelers 1982.* MMWR 31, Atlanta, 1982.
11. CDC: *Sexually Transmitted Diseases Treatment Guidelines 1982.* MMWR 31, Atlanta, 1982.
12. Clark DW, MacMahon B: *Preventive and Community Medicine,* 2nd ed. Little, Brown, Boston, 1981.

13. Clays HH: *Handbook on Environmental Health,* 14th ed (Revised by F. G. Davies.) H. K. Lewis, London, 1977.

14. Cralley LV, Atkins PR: *Industrial Environmental Health,* 2nd ed. Academic Press, New York, 1975.

15. Fisher AA: *Contact Dermatitis.* Lea & Febiger, Philadelphia, 1967.

16. Fitzpatrick TB, Eisen AZ, Wolff K, Freedberg IM, Austen KF: *Dermatology in General Medicine,* 2nd ed. McGraw-Hill, New York, 1979.

17. Fox JP, Hall CE, Elveback LR: *Epidemiology: Man and Disease.* Macmillan, London, 1972.

18. Freedman D, Pisani R, Purves R: *Statistics.* W. W. Norton, New York, 1978.

19. Gardner AW: *Current Approaches to Occupational Health — 2,* John Wright & Sons, Bristol, England, 1982.

20. Grant M: *Handbook of Community Health,* 3rd ed. Lea & Febiger, Philadelphia, 1981.

21. Hamilton A, Hardy HL: *Industrial Toxicology,* 4th ed. (Edited by Asher J. Finkel.) PSG Inc., Boston, 1983.

22. Hanlon JJ, Pickett GE: *Public Health: Administration and Practice,* 7th ed. C. V. Mosby, St. Louis, 1979.

23. Hobson W: *Theory and Practice of Public Health,* 5th ed. Oxford University Press, Oxford, England, 1979.

24. Howe GM: *A World Geography of Human Disease.* Academic Press, London, 1977.

25. Howe GM, Loraine JA: *Environmental Medicine,* 2nd ed. William Heinemann Medical Books, London, 1980.

26. Ipsen J, Feigl P: *Bancroft's Introduction to Biostatistics,* 2nd ed. Harper & Row, New York, 1970.

27. Kilbourne ED, Smillie WG: *Human Ecology and Public Health,* 4th ed. Macmillan, London, 1969.

28. Leaverton PE: *A Review of Biostatistics.* Little, Brown, Boston, 1978.

29. Lilienfeld AM: *Foundations of Epidemiology.* Oxford University Press, New York, 1976.

30. Lucas AO, Gilles HM: *A Short Textbook of Preventive Medicine for the Tropics.* Hodder & Stoughton, London, 1981.

31. MacKie RM: *Clinical Dermatology.* Oxford University Press, Oxford, England, 1981.

32. Mackinson FW, Stricoff RS, Partride LJ: *Occupational Health Guidelines for Chemical Hazards.* U.S. Department of HHS (NIOSH/OSHA) Publication No. 81-123, Washington, D.C., 1981.

33. MacMahon B, Pugh TF, et al: *Epidemiology.* Little, Brown, Boston, 1970.

34. Maibach HI, Gellin GA: *Occupational and Industrial Dermatology.* Year Book Medical Publishers, Chicago, 1982.

35. Manson-Bahr PEG, Apted FIC: *Manson's Tropical Disease,* 18th ed. Macmillan, New York, 1982.

36. Mason TJ, McKay FW, et al: *Atlas of Cancer Mortalities for U.S. Counties 1950-1969.* U.S. Department of HEW, Epidemiology Branch, DHEW Publication No. (NIH) 75-780, Washington, D.C.

37. Maxcy-Rosenau KR: *Public Health and Preventive Medicine,* 11th ed. (Edited by John M. Last.) Appleton-Century-Crofts, New York, 1980.

38. Mayers MR: *Occupational Health, Hazards of the Work Environment.* Williams & Wilkins, Baltimore, 1969.

39. Monson RR: *Occupational Epidemiology.* CRC Press, Boca Raton, Fla., 1980.

40. OSHA: *Report of the Advisory Committee on Cutaneous Hazards to Assistant Secretary of Labor,* OSHA, Washington, D.C., 1978.

41. Parkes WR: *Occupational Lung Disorders,* 2nd ed. Butterworth, London, 1982.

42. Pene P, Bourgeade A, Delmont J: *Medicine Tropicale en Pays Tempères.* Doin, Paris, 1982.

43. Peñalver RA: *Manganese Poisoning.* Proceedings of the Eighth Asian Conference on Occupational Health, Tokyo, 1976.

44. Petrie A: *Lecture Notes on Medical Statistics.* Blackwell, Oxford, England, 1978.

45. Proctor NH, Hughes JP: *Chemical Hazards of the Workplace.* Lippincott, Philadelphia, 1978.

46. Randel HW: *Aerospace Medicine.* Williams & Wilkins, Baltimore, 1971.

47. Rimm AA, Hartz AJ, et al: *Basic Biostatistics in Medicine.* Appleton-Century-Crofts, New York, 1980.

48. Rotschild HR: *Biocultural Aspects of Disease.* Academic Press, New York, 1981.

49. Sandstead HH, Carter JP, Darby WJ: How To Diagnose Nutritional Deficiencies. *Nutrition Today* 4:2-12, 1969.

50. Shaw CR: *Prevention of Occupational Cancer.* CRC Press, Boca Raton, Fla., 1981.

51. Shilling CW: *Radiation, Use and Control in Industrial Application.* Grune & Stratton, New York, 1960.

52. Solomons B: *Lecture Notes on Dermatology,* 4th ed. Blackwell, Oxford, England, 1977.

53. Spencer PS, Schaumburg HH: *Experimental and Clinical Neurotoxicology.* Williams & Wilkins, Baltimore, 1980.

54. Stahl SM, Hennes JD: *Reading and Understanding Applied Statistics,* 2nd ed. C. V. Mosby, St. Louis, 1980.

55. Stokinger HE: Industrial Air Standards: Theory and Practice. *Journal of Occupational Medicine* 15:429-431, 1973.

56. Swinscow TDV: *Statistics at Square One*. British Medical Association, London, 1978.

57. Tartakow IJ, Vorperian JH: *Foodborne and Waterborne Disease*. AVI Publishing Co., Westport, Conn., 1981.

58. Tyrer FH, Lee K: *A Synopsis of Occupational Medicine*. John Wright & Sons, Bristol, England, 1979.

59. U.S. Department of HEW: *Syphilis: A Synopsis*. U.S. Government Printing Office, Publication No. 1660, Washington, D.C., 1968.

60. Waldron HA: *Lecture Notes on Occupational Medicine,* 2nd ed. Blackwell, Oxford, England, 1979.

61. Waldron HA, Harrington JM: *Occupational Hygiene: An Introductory Text*. Blackwell, Oxford, England, 1980.

62. Wisdom A: *A Colour Atlas of Venereology*. Wolfe Medical Books, London, 1973.

63. Zenz C: *Occupational Medicine, Principles and Practical Applications*. Year Book Medical Publishers, Chicago, 1975.

CHAPTER ONE

Biostatistics and Population Dynamics

Directions: Each of the questions or incomplete statements below is followed by five suggested answers or completions. Select the BEST answer in each case.

1. The crude birth rate is determined by dividing the number of live births reported during a given time interval by the

   A. number of married women 15 to 44 years old
   B. number of women in their childbearing years (usually taken as 15–44)
   C. total female population
   D. estimated midinterval population
   E. number of live births and stillbirths during the same time interval

2. The maternal mortality rate comprises death due to

   A. complications of delivery
   B. complications of pregnancy
   C. abortion
   D. complications of the puerperium
   E. all of the above

3. Which of the following is the best reflection of the levels of sanitation and nutrition of a country?

   A. crude death rate
   B. fetal mortality rate
   C. neonatal mortality rate
   D. infant mortality rate
   E. case fatality rate

4. A decrease in the prevalence of a disease may be interpreted as being a result of

   A. a reduction in the incidence
   B. a more rapid cure
   C. increased migration of affected persons from the community
   D. a shorter life span of affected persons
   E. all of the above

5. If the average duration of a disease is three years and its incidence rate is 10 per 1,000, the prevalence rate will be

   A. 3 × 1,000
   B. 6 × 1,000
   C. 9 × 1,000
   D. 30 × 1,000
   E. 90 × 1,000

6. What does the following formula represent?

   $$\frac{\text{Observed number of deaths}}{\text{Expected number of deaths}} \times 100 =$$

   A. crude death rate
   B. age-specific death rate
   C. cause-specific death rate
   D. standardized mortality ratio (SMR)
   E. none of the above

7. In this set of data: 35, 24, 15, 19, 6, 11, 12, the median is

   A. 23
   B. 15
   C. 61
   D. 20
   E. 11

8. In this set of data: 13, 27, 29, 11, 5, 5, the median is

   A. 18
   B. 5
   C. 12
   D. 24
   E. 45

9. The standard deviation always indicates the scatter of the individual measurements around their

   A. mode
   B. median
   C. midrange
   D. arithmetic mean
   E. unweighted mean

10. If the mean weight in a group of 50 men is 170 lb, with a standard deviation of 15 lb,

    A. 95% of individual weights fall between 155 and 185 lb
    B. 66% of individual weights fall between 140 and 200 lb
    C. 95% of individual weights fall between 140 and 200 lb
    D. no individual weight is more than 185 lb
    E. no individual weight is less than 155 lb

11. In all distributions, the fiftieth percentile is equivalent to the

    A. mean
    B. mode
    C. median
    D. range
    E. standard deviation

12. What would be the likelihood of throwing a 2 or a 5 in one throw of a die?

    A. 2:5
    B. 1:6
    C. 1:3
    D. 1:36
    E. 1:12

13. What is the probability of rolling a 1, a 2, and a 5, in that order, from three rolls of a die?

    A. 1:216
    B. 1:36
    C. 1:8
    D. 1:18
    E. impossible to calculate because information is insufficient

14. The probability of contracting "illness A" during one's lifetime is approximately 0.006, and the probability of contracting "illness B" is approximately 0.02. If these two events are independent, the probability of one person contracting both illnesses during his lifetime is approximately

    A. 0.00013
    B. 0.00026
    C. 0.00012
    D. 0.00014
    E. 0.00035

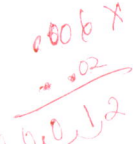

15. "Expectation of life" means

    A. the number of persons surviving to age X
    B. the number of persons dying between age X and age X + 1 (between one age and the next)
    C. the probability of surviving from age X to age X + 1
    D. the probability of dying between age X and age X + 1
    E. the average length of life to be lived beyond age X

16. In general, life expectancy is greater for females than for males in

    A. age group 0–4 years
    B. age group 5–9 years
    C. age group 20–24 years
    D. age group 40–44 years
    E. all of the above

17. Which of the following constitute(s) the leading cause of death in the United States?

    A. malignant neoplasms
    B. arteriosclerosis
    C. bronchitis, emphysema, and asthma
    D. diseases of the heart
    E. homicide

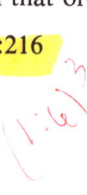

18. Which of the following is *not* among the five leading causes of death for children one to four years old in the United States?

    A. accidents
    B. congenital malformations
    C. influenza and pneumonia
    D. malignant neoplasms
    E. gastritis, enteritis, and colitis

19. Which of the following is *not* among the five leading causes of death for children five to 14 years old in the United States?

    A. accidents
    B. malignant neoplasms
    C. congenital malformations
    D. cardiovascular and renal disease
    E. tuberculosis

20. Mortality drops to its lowest level in which of the following age groups?

    A. 1-4 years
    B. 5-9 years
    C. 10-14 years
    D. 15-19 years
    E. 20-24 years

21. The greatest decline in mortality rates in the United States in the last half century has been observed in which of the following age groups?

    A. 1-4 years
    B. 5-9 years
    C. 10-14 years
    D. 15-19 years
    E. 20-24 years

22. Fatal home accidents are most likely to occur in the

    A. kitchen
    B. bedroom
    C. bathroom
    D. swimming pool
    E. garden

23. Which of the following is the single most important determinant in disease morbidity and mortality?

    A. sex
    B. race and ethnic background
    C. genetic makeup
    D. age
    E. birth order

24. In general, seasonal variation is *not* a prominent feature in the incidence of

    A. chronic diseases
    B. Rocky Mountain spotted fever
    C. equine encephalitis
    D. accidents
    E. poliomyelitis

25. Screening programs, through suitable available tests, may uncover all of the following conditions *except*

    A. glaucoma
    B. rheumatoid arthritis
    C. diabetes mellitus
    D. high blood pressure
    E. hearing disorders

26. Which is the most common cause of blindness in the United States?

    A. ophthalmia neonatorum
    B. congenital syphilis
    C. retrolental fibroplasia
    D. senile cataracts
    E. trachoma

27. The principal factor in the occurrence of retrolental fibroplasia is

    A. hypervitaminosis A
    B. gonococcal infection
    C. lack of illumination
    D. vibration
    E. overuse of oxygen in premature infants

28. Age-adjusted death rates for coronary heart disease are highest in

    A. Portugal
    B. Spain
    C. Italy
    D. the United States
    E. Japan

29. Which of the following is probably the most common single risk indicator in the development of coronary heart disease?

    A. genetic inheritance
    B. diabetes mellitus
    C. behavior pattern
    D. hypertension
    E. sex

30. Which of the following is the most frequent kidney disease leading to transplantation?

    A. glomerulonephritis
    B. pyelonephritis
    C. polycystic disease
    D. nephrosclerosis
    E. congenital kidney disease

31. In the United States more than 60% of all urinary stones are composed of

    A. uric acid
    B. magnesium ammonium phosphate
    C. silicates
    D. calcium oxalate
    E. cystine

32. All of the following are characteristics of hepatolenticular degeneration (Wilson's disease) except

    A. decrease in the concentration of serum ceruloplasmin and total serum copper
    B. aminoaciduria
    C. serum phosphate and serum uric acid may be decreased
    D. tremor and rigidity, particularly in early adult life
    E. has been described as a result of chronic industrial exposure to copper

33. Hepatolenticular degeneration (Wilson's disease) is characterized by

    A. pigmentation of the outer margin of the cornea in the form of a smoky brownish ring (Kayser-Fleischer ring)
    B. increased urinary copper excretion
    C. increased deposition of copper in all organs
    D. penicillamine being the drug of choice
    E. all of the above

34. The prevalence of which of the following handicaps is higher in children under 21 years old in the United States?

    A. emotional problems
    B. mental retardation
    C. orthopedic problems
    D. speech defects
    E. cardiac defects

35. Among patients hospitalized for mental illness, which of the following is the most common condition?

    A. manic depression
    B. schizophrenia
    C. alcoholic psychosis
    D. syphilitic psychosis
    E. mental diseases of the senium

36. Which of the following have the highest annual suicide rate in the Unites States?

    A. military personnel
    B. physicians
    C. teachers
    D. lawyers
    E. miners

37. Which of the following inherited metabolic disorders is associated with mental retardation?

    A. congenital thyroid deficiency
    B. galactosemia
    C. maple syrup urine disease
    D. homocysteinuria
    E. all of the above

38. All of the following statements about multiple sclerosis are true except

    A. no preventive measures are known
    B. it is more common in the Southern Hemisphere
    C. it is characterized clinically by remissions and recurrences over a period of many years
    D. the cause of the disease is unknown
    E. an increase in familial occurrence has long been recognized

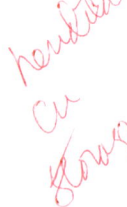

39. Intravenous injection of which of the following drugs may be used to distinguish myasthenic crisis (which improves) from overtreatment intoxication (no change or further weakens) in myasthenic patients under treatment?

   A. pyridostigmine bromide (Mestinon)
   B. neostigmine bromide (Prostigmin bromide)
   C. ambenonium chloride (Mytelase chloride)
   D. edrophonium chloride (Tensilon)
   E. Prednisone

40. The most deadly complication of narcotic addiction is

   A. viral hepatitis
   B. pneumonia
   C. bacterial endocarditis
   D. overdose
   E. syphilis

41. If present rates continue, the percentage of Americans now living who will eventually have cancer is

   A. 5%
   B. 10%
   C. 15%
   D. 20%
   E. 33%

42. According to the World Health Organization (WHO), the percentage of all cancers caused by environmental factors is

   A. between 75 and 80%
   B. between 55 and 65%
   C. between 35 and 45%
   D. between 15 and 25%
   E. between 5 and 10%

43. Which type of cancer is responsible for the majority of male deaths?

   A. stomach cancer
   B. respiratory cancer
   C. pancreatic cancer
   D. leukemia
   E. bladder cancer

44. A low incidence among Jewish women has been observed for which of the following?

   A. cancer of the esophagus
   B. cancer of the skin
   C. cancer of the cervix
   D. cancer of the breast
   E. cancer of the bladder

45. An epidemiologic description of the woman at increased risk of breast cancer would include all of the following *except*

   A. early age at menarche
   B. late age at first live birth
   C. obesity
   D. being a native-born Japanese woman as contrasted with being a U.S. white or black woman
   E. high socioeconomic status

46. The cancer or Delaney Clause of the Food Additive Amendment Act of 1958 applies to

   A. air pollution
   B. water pollution
   C. food additives
   D. radiation control
   E. noise control

47. At the time of Christ the population of the world had reached about 250 million. The current figure is about

   A. 500 million people
   B. 800 million people
   C. one billion people
   D. two billion people
   E. four billion people

48. Over all, the world's population is currently increasing at the rate of over

   A. 50,000 per day
   B. 100,000 per day
   C. 150,000 per day
   D. 200,000 per day
   E. 200,000 per month

49. The rate of population increase varies in different parts of the world. The highest annual increase (1975) occurred in

   A. Europe

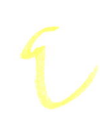

A. North America
B. Asia
C. Africa
E. Latin America

50. In the United States a census is taken every

    A. year
    B. three years
    C. leap year
    D. five years
    E. 10 years

51. The number of years required to double the population at a 3% annual rate of increase is

    A. 18
    B. 20
    C. 23
    D. 28
    E. 35

52. The annual rate of increase required to double the population in 18 years is

    A. 4.0%
    B. 3.5%
    C. 3.0%
    D. 2.5%
    E. 2.0%

53. Of the following, which is the most effective contraceptive method?

    A. hormonal contraception — "the pill"
    B. intrauterine devices (IUDs)
    C. vaginal foam tablets
    D. condom
    E. rhythm method

54. Which of the following are responsible for more than 50% of the cases of acute conditions causing absenteeism in the United States?

    A. digestive conditions
    B. respiratory conditions
    C. skin diseases
    D. occupational injuries
    E. nonoccupational injuries

55. Currently, in the United States, approximately how many work days are lost, per worker per year, as a result of illness or injury?

    A. two
    B. four
    C. six
    D. eight
    E. 10

56. Which of the following statements referring to expert witness is *incorrect*?

    A. In general, any licensed physician is considered to qualify as an expert witness in controversies dealing with medical questions.
    B. Certification by medical specialty board is necessary.
    C. The physician, as expert witness, may give an opinion even if he never before saw either litigant.
    D. The physician may give an opinion even if he never before observed a similar case.
    E. Compensation can never be contingent on the winning of the suit by the person for whom the physician appears as a witness.

57. More than 40% of the total personal health care dollar in the United States in 1980 went to

    A. hospital care
    B. physicians' services
    C. dentists' services
    D. nursing home care
    E. drug and drug sundries

58. In the United States the most hazardous time for a newborn child is the

    A. first summer after birth
    B. first week of life
    C. second week of life
    D. second month of life
    E. first winter after birth

59. The most important factor in deaths occurring during the first week of life is

    A. prematurity
    B. congenital malformations

C. influenza
D. pneumonia
E. gastrointestinal disorders

60. Approximately what percentage of all births in the United States are premature?

    A. 1%
    B. 2.5%
    C. 3.8%
    D. 6.5%
    E. 8.8%

61. In the United States, since 1935 the proportion of hospital deliveries has increased from less than 40% to more than

    A. 55%
    B. 65%
    C. 75%
    D. 85%
    E. 95%

62. The frequency of twin confinements among white births in the United States is approximately

    A. 1%
    B. 2%
    C. 3%
    D. 4%
    E. 5%

63. Which of the following does *not* appear to be related in any way with genetic factors?

    A. fibrocystic disease of the pancreas
    B. hemophilia
    C. cancer of the breast
    D. measles
    E. gout

Directions: Each group of questions below consists of five lettered headings followed by a list of numbered words or phrases. For each numbered word or phrase select the one heading that is most closely related to it.

Questions 64 through 68

A. Cause-specific death rate
B. Incidence
C. Crude death rate
D. Prevalence
E. Age-specific death rate

64. 8.8 deaths per 1,000 population per year
65. 19.96 asthmatics per 100,000 population
66. 31.4 deaths at ages 65–74 per 1,000 population aged 65–74 per year
67. 181.6 deaths from cancer per 100,000 population per year
68. in an employed population of average age 45, 5% of the workers have diabetes

Questions 69 through 73

A. Perinatal mortality
B. Early neonatal mortality
C. Postneonatal mortality
D. Late neonatal mortality
E. Neonatal mortality

69. deaths under four weeks of age
70. deaths under one week of age
71. deaths between one and four weeks of age
72. deaths over four weeks and under one year of age
73. stillbirths and deaths under one week of age

Questions 74 through 78

A. Crude death rate
B. Maternal mortality rate
C. Cause-specific death rate
D. Age-specific death rate
E. None of the above

74. number of deaths assigned to causes related to pregnancy during a given time interval, divided by the total number of women who became pregnant during the year
75. number of deaths assigned to a specific cause during a given time interval, divided by the number of new cases of that disease reported during the same time interval

76. number of deaths in a certain age group, divided by the average population in the same age group during the same period

77. total number of deaths reported during a given time interval, divided by the estimated mid-interval population

78. number of deaths under one year of age reported during a given time interval, divided by the number of births reported during the same time interval

Questions 79 through 83

Set of data: 7, 3, 4, 6, 1, 6, 7, 6, 5

A. 4
B. 6
C. 5
D. 2
E. 3

79. midrange
80. range
81. median
82. mode
83. arithmetic mean

Questions 84 through 88

A. Range
B. Mode
C. Arithmetic mean
D. Median
E. Midrange

84. the middle ranking number of a set of observations
85. the simple average of a set of observations
86. the most frequently occurring value in a set of observations
87. the difference between the largest and smallest value in a set of observations
88. the arithmetic mean of the smallest and largest observations

Questions 89 through 91

In a normal curve

A. 99.72%
B. 95.44%
C. 72.54%
D. 68.26%
E. 33%

of the area will be

89. included between +1 and −1 standard deviation
90. included between +3 and −3 standard deviation
91. included between +2 and −2 standard deviation

Questions 92 through 96

A. Accidents
B. Malignant neoplasms
C. Diseases of the heart
D. Cerebrovascular disease
E. Diabetes mellitus

Leading cause of death:

92. age group: one to four years
93. age group: five to 14 years
94. age group: 15–24 years
95. age group: 25–44 years
96. age group: 45–64 years

Questions 97 through 101

A. Barbiturates
B. Codeine
C. LSD (lysergic acid diethylamide)
D. Heroin
E. Amphetamines

97. dilated pupils, excitability, rapid and unclear speech, dry mouth, continued use results in increased pulse and blood pressure, hallucinations, psychoses — medical use: weight reduction

98. constricted pupils, relaxation, slurred speech, flushing of skin or face, continued use results in scars or abscesses at injection points

99. dilated pupils, increased pulse rate and blood pressure, hallucinogen, continued use may result in psychoses, possible chromosomal breakdown and organic brain damage

100. pinpoint pupils, drowsiness, continued use develops tolerance to drug, prescribed orally to relieve pain and coughing

101. similar to alcohol intoxication, uncoordination, tremors, depressant, continued use results in depressed pulse and blood pressure, possible convulsions — medical use: for sedation and sleep

Questions 102 through 106

    A. Buccal (cheek) cancer
    B. Cancer of the nasopharynx
    C. Skin cancer
    D. Cancer of the stomach
    E. Cancer of the esophagus

102. The highest incidence in the world is found in eastern Australia. Hydrocarbons, x-rays, and sun radiation are potent causes.

103. This form of cancer occurs only where a concoction of various ingredients is wrapped in a pan of leaf and chewed. This custom is practiced in south India and New Guinea.

104. Epstein-Barr virus (EBV). Chinese populations in southeast Asia have maximal prevalences of this tumor.

105. The incidence in Puerto Rico is among the highest in the world. Common in China. Alcohol has been incriminated.

106. The highest rates in the world occur in Japan and Korea. For unknown reasons, marked decline in the United States. Pernicious anemia.

Biostatistics and Population Dynamics

Questions 107 through 111

    A. Cancer of the liver
    B. Bladder cancer
    C. Melanoma
    D. Breast cancer
    E. Stomach cancer

107. May have an environmental factor in common with cancers of the large intestine.

108. Deaths occur predominantly in the southern United States. Sunlight may be a major factor.

109. High rates in the North Central states of the United States (corresponding closely with the geographic concentration of persons with ancestors from Austria, the Soviet Union, and Scandinavia).

110. For males, clusters of excessive mortality occur in New Jersey, New York City, and urban areas around the Great Lakes. In Salem County (N.J.), one-fourth of the work force is employed in chemical and allied industries.

111. High incidence among the Bantu in Africa.

Questions 112 through 116

    A. Intestinal cancer
    B. Primary liver cancer
    C. Bladder cancer
    D. Cancer of the mouth
    E. Cancer of the gallbladder

112. Uncommon in western countries. Associated with a toxin (aflatoxin) produced by a fungus (*Aspergillus flavus*), and also with hepatitis B.

113. Multiple polyposis.

114. Unusually frequent in Egypt and other areas where schistosomiasis is prevalent.

115. High rate of cholelithiasis.

116. Plummer-Vinson syndrome.

Questions 117 through 121

A. Benzene
B. Vinyl chloride monomer
C. Radium dial painters
D. Chimney sweeps
E. Wood dust

117. osteosarcoma
118. leukemia
119. angiosarcoma of the liver
120. cancer of the scrotum
121. nasal cavity and nasal sinuses cancer

Questions 122 through 126

A. Lung cancer
B. Bladder cancer
C. Skin cancer
D. Leukemia
E. Cancer of the prostate

122. radiologists
123. xeroderma pigmentosum
124. dyestuff workers
125. nickel refiners
126. chromate production workers

Questions 127 through 131

A. Cancer of the prostate
B. Thyroid cancer
C. Liver cancer
D. Carcinoma of the vagina in adolescent girls
E. Leukemia

127. mothers treated during pregnancy with diethylstilbestrol (DES)
128. chloramphenicol
129. therapeutic radiation for ankylosing spondylitis
130. Cytoxan for rheumatoid arthritis
131. irradiation to the neck in childhood for thymic enlargement

Questions 132 through 136

A. Thorotrast administration
B. Fluoroscopic examination of the chest
C. Herpes simplex virus of the genital tract (HSV-2)
D. "Mule spinners"
E. "Pipe fitters"

132. breast cancer
133. angiosarcoma of the liver
134. cancer of the cervix
135. cancer of the scrotum
136. mesothelioma

Questions 137 through 141

A. Maternal age
B. Paternal age
C. Family size
D. Birth order
E. None of the above

137. hypertrophic pyloric stenosis
138. Down's syndrome
139. erythroblastosis fetalis
140. dizygotic twinning
141. patent ductus arteriosus

Questions 142 through 146

Maternal medication

A. Chloramphenicol
B. Tetracyclines
C. Magnesium sulfate
D. Sulfasalazine (Azulfidine)
E. Streptomycin sulfate

Fetal or neonatal effect

142. kernicterus
143. Grey syndrome

144. hearing loss (eighth nerve damage)

145. temporary depression of bone growth, tooth enamel damage

146. may suppress skeletal muscle activity in the neonate

Questions 147 through 151

Maternal medication

A. Diazepam
B. Androgens
C. Amphetamines
D. Vitamin D (large dose)
E. Dicumarol

Fetal or neonatal effect

147. masculinization of female fetus

148. birth defects, hemorrhage, fetal death

149. low Apgar scores, apnea, and feeding problems (the floppy infant syndrome)

150. hyperglycemia, agitation

151. supravalvular aortic stenosis, tetany

Questions 152 through 156

Maternal medication

A. Phenobarbital
B. Phenothiazines
C. Mepivacaine
D. Reserpine
E. Propylthiouracil

Fetal or neonatal effect

152. bleeding

153. goiter, hypothyroidism

154. nasal congestion, drowsiness, cyanosis, anorexia

155. bradycardia, central nervous system depression

156. prolonged extrapyramidal effects

Directions: Each set of lettered headings below is followed by a list of numbered words or phrases. For each numbered word or phrase select

A. if the item is associated with A only
B. if the item is associated with B only
C. if the item is associated with both A and B
D. if the item is associated with neither A nor B

Questions 157 through 161

A. Incidence rate
B. Prevalence rate
C. Both
D. Neither

157. number of new cases of disease per unit of population per unit of time

158. number of existent cases of disease per unit of population

159. a static measure of disease frequency

160. useful for studying disease causation and the evaluation of preventive measures

161. children with a birth defect divided by the total children born (birth defect rate)

Questions 162 through 166

A. Sensitivity
B. Specificity
C. Both
D. Neither

162. ability to identify correctly those who have the disease

163. calculated by dividing the number of disease-free individuals who have a negative test by the total number of persons tested who do not have the disease

164. indicates the strength of an association

165. denotes the uniqueness of an association

166. component of the validity of a test; in actuality, values of 100% seldom, if ever, occur

Questions 167 through 171

A. Prospective epidemiologic studies
B. Retrospective epidemiologic studies
C. Both
D. Neither

167. the purpose of this type of study is to identify the presence of an association between a risk factor and disease

168. "negative predictive" value of a negative association"

169. "sensitivity"

170. study is usually long in duration and relatively expensive

171. relates events in an "after-before" sequence

Questions 172 through 176

A. Validity
B. Reliability
C. Both
D. Neither

172. synonymous with accuracy

173. refers to how consistently a measure measures whatever is being measured

174. used synonymously for precision

175. refers to whether what is claimed to be measured is in fact measured

176. a characteristic of measurement

Questions 177 through 181

A. Developing countries
B. Economically developed countries
C. Both
D. Neither

177. a triangular broad-based pattern population pyramid

178. high maternal mortality rate

179. population growth rates may exceed 3.5% per year

180. life expectancy and the median age of the population are both high, indicating an "older population"

181. high prevalence of coronary heart disease

Questions 182 through 186

A. Blue Cross Health Insurance
B. Blue Shield Health Insurance
C. Both
D. Neither

182. essentially a nonprofit medical care prepayment insurance plan

183. with minor exceptions, devoted to provide benefits for hospitalization

184. hospital care for indigents

185. covers hospital costs and physician services for industrially compensable cases

186. provides for psychiatric services

Directions: For each of the incomplete statements below, ONE or MORE of the completions given is correct. In each case select

A. if only 1, 2, and 3 are correct
B. if only 1 and 3 are correct
C. if only 2 and 4 are correct
D. if only 4 is correct
E. if all are correct

Questions 187 through 226

187. "Actual" suicide rates in the United States are

   1. higher among men than among women
   2. lower among native-born Americans than among immigrants
   3. higher in central cities than in the suburbs
   4. lower among blacks than among whites

188. Chronic alcoholism is

   1. more frequent among men than among women
   2. a major cause of absenteeism

3. more frequent in urban than in rural areas
4. a major cause of occupational accidents

189. Withdrawal syndromes can be seen following prolonged
    1. morphine use
    2. alcohol ingestion
    3. heroin use
    4. barbiturate ingestion

190. Which of the following may be associated with an increased risk of lung cancer?
    1. coke-oven workers
    2. workers engaged in smelting and refining copper, lead, and zinc ores
    3. cigarette smoking
    4. uranium miners

191. Which of the following cancers are considered to be asbestos-related?
    1. lung cancer
    2. cancer of the throat
    3. mesothelioma
    4. cancer of the stomach

192. Which of the following have been found to be associated with elevated rates of cervical cancer?
    1. lower socioeconomic status
    2. early frequent sexual activity
    3. multiple pregnancies
    4. genetic predisposition

193. Which of the following is (are) true of Burkitt's lymphoma?
    1. the peak incidence is found in the four- to eight-year-old group
    2. same geographical distribution as that of the anopheles mosquitoes
    3. associated with the Epstein-Barr (EB) virus
    4. the tumor responds well, often dramatically, to chemotherapy

194. For which of the following is the mortality higher among women than men?
    1. thyroid cancer
    2. gallbladder cancer
    3. breast cancer
    4. laryngeal cancer

195. For which of the following forms of cancer is incidence directly related to fat consumption?
    1. cancer of the prostate
    2. breast cancer
    3. cancer of the endometrium
    4. intestinal cancer

196. The American Board of Preventive Medicine certifies competence in the field(s) of
    1. public health
    2. aerospace medicine
    3. occupational medicine
    4. general preventive medicine

197. Prematurity may be associated with
    1. toxemia of pregnancy
    2. placenta praevia
    3. hypertension
    4. multiple pregnancies

198. Which of the following has (have) been implicated in the genesis of congenital malformations?
    1. infectious agents
    2. chemical agents
    3. physical agents
    4. trauma

199. The crude birth rate
    1. is the most frequently quoted fertility rate
    2. is usually computed on a residence basis
    3. is defined as the number of live births per 1,000 population during a year
    4. measures the risk of childbearing

200. The crude mortality or death rate
    1. attempts to measure the rate at which a population is dying
    2. if calculated on an annual basis, the denominator will be the estimated population as of July 1st of the same year

3. has an accuracy dependent on the completeness with which deaths have been reported
4. has a denominator that is the number of deaths reported during a given time period, usually a year

201. The denominator of the maternal mortality rate includes

1. all women having a stillbirth
2. all women having a miscarriage
3. all women having an abortion
4. each live-born child in multiple pregnancies

202. Incidence rate(s) include the

1. birth rate
2. attack rate
3. mortality rate
4. cure rate

203. Attack rates are characterized by which of the following?

1. number of cases of a disease that develop in a population during some fixed time period
2. concept of incidence rate
3. units of prevalence rate
4. used in infectious disease epidemiology

204. A measure of central tendency is the

1. mode
2. arithmetic mean
3. median
4. range

205. A measure of dispersion is the

1. range
2. percentiles
3. semi-interquartile range
4. standard deviation

206. Which of the following statements about the standard deviation is (are) correct?

1. states how far away numbers on a list are from their average

2. most entries on the list will be somewhere around one standard deviation away from the average
3. very few entries will be more than two or three standard deviations away from the average
4. uses every observation

207. With respect to percentiles,

1. they are numbers that divide a distribution, or the area of a histogram, into 100 parts of equal area
2. the tenth percentile exceeds 10% of the observations
3. the tenth percentile is exceeded by 90% of the observations
4. they provide a way of describing the variation of frequency distribution regardless of the shape of the distribution

208. With respect to quartiles,

1. they are the percentiles that divide the distribution into quarters
2. the 25th percentile is the third quartile
3. the 50th percentile is the second quartile
4. the 75th percentile is the first quartile

209. Discrete variable is a term that could be applied to

1. number of tablets in a bottle
2. number of pregnancies
3. population expressed in number of individuals
4. blood pressure

210. Continuous variable is a term that could be applied to

1. height expressed in centimeters
2. age expressed in years
3. weight expressed in pounds
4. number of hospital admissions

211. In statistics, the term population means

1. objects
2. events
3. observations
4. people

212. Random samples can be obtained only by use of a formal randomization device such as

   1. using a table of random numbers
   2. pulling numbers out of a hat
   3. tossing coins
   4. asking for volunteers

213. The correlation coefficient

   1. is a measure of the degree of association found between two characteristics in a series of observations (on the assumption that the relationship between the two characteristics is adequately described by a straight line)
   2. its value must lie between +1 and −1
   3. a plus (+) sign shows that an upward movement of one characteristic is accompanied by an upward movement in the other
   4. a negative (−) sign denotes no association whatever between the two characteristics

214. The correlation coefficient is a pure number, without units. It is unaffected by

   1. interchanging the two variables
   2. adding the same number to all the values of one variable
   3. multiplying all the values of one variable by the same positive number
   4. interchanging the last two values for the second variable

215. Among the 10 leading causes of death in the United States is (are)

   1. diseases of the heart
   2. malignant neoplasms
   3. cerebrovascular disease
   4. accidents

216. Which of the following statements about home accidents is (are) true?

   1. their frequency approaches half of all accidents
   2. among men the highest home injury rate occurs in the highest income group
   3. falls are the most frequent cause of death
   4. the kitchen is the locale of the highest percentage of all accidents

217. Diseases that occur primarily among men include

   1. cholecystitis
   2. duodenal ulcer
   3. thyrotoxicosis
   4. coronary heart disease

218. Which of the following diseases occur(s) primarily among women?

   1. gout
   2. cirrhosis
   3. arteriosclerotic heart disease
   4. diabetes mellitus

219. Which of the following diseases occur(s) primarily among whites?

   1. tuberculosis
   2. hypertension
   3. sarcoidosis
   4. pyloric stenosis of infancy

220. Which of the following diseases is (are) more frequent (age-adjusted rates) among urban than among rural residents?

   1. cancer of the lung
   2. cirrhosis of the liver
   3. arteriosclerotic heart disease
   4. St. Louis encephalitis

221. Which of the following factors is (are) believed to contribute to the cause of ischemic heart disease?

   1. high intake of fat
   2. smoking
   3. obesity and diabetes
   4. exercise

222. The usual age at first hospital admission is between 16 and 35 years for

   1. manic depressive psychosis
   2. alcoholic psychosis
   3. senile psychosis
   4. schizophrenia

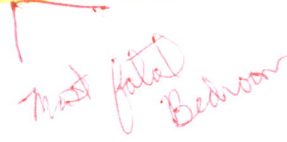

223. Which of the following diseases occur(s) more frequently among lower than among upper socioeconomic groups?
    1. schizophrenia
    2. neuroses
    3. mild mental retardation
    4. manic depressive psychoses

224. Major advances have been made in the prevention of mental disease caused by
    1. syphilis
    2. pellagra
    3. lead poisoning
    4. senile arteriosclerosis

225. There is no significant difference between the sexes with respect to the incidence of
    1. mental deficiency
    2. alcoholic psychoses
    3. senile psychoses
    4. personality disorders (nonalcoholic)

226. Which of the following disorders is (are) more frequent among women?
    1. schizophrenia
    2. psychoneuroses
    3. manic depression
    4. involutional psychoses

Answers and Explanations: Biostatistics and Population Dynamics

1. **D.** The birth rate for a given community for a calendar year is defined as the ratio of live births occurring among the residents of that community during the calendar year to the population at midyear, and the results are quoted as live births per 1,000 population per year. (17:127)

2. **E.** The maternal mortality rate is expressed as deaths from maternal causes per thousand total births, live and still, during the same year. (23:23)

3. **D.** The infant mortality rate represents the number of deaths of infants under one year of age divided by the live births in the community in the year of study. Infant death rates closely correlate with socioeconomic development, which includes conditions that affect the level of nutrition, sanitation, and hygiene. (12:38)

4. **E.** In general, if the incidence rate increases, the prevalence rate increases. If the "cure rate" of a disease increases, the prevalence rate decreases. If the mortality rate of a disease increases, the prevalence rate decreases. (35:29)

5. **D.** The prevalence rate equals the incidence rate times the average duration of the disease. (29:118)

6. **D.** Standardized mortality ratio: relation between the number of deaths at all ages observed in a given population and the number of deaths that would have occurred in that population if in each age (and sex) group it had been exposed to some selected standard rates. (50:62)

7. **B.** The median is the middle of a series of values arranged in order of magnitude. In this series of seven values—6, 11, 12, 15, 19, 24, 35—the median is the fourth value, 15, since half of the values exceed it and half are below it. (3:101)

8. **C.** In this series of six (even) values—5, 5, 11, 13, 27, 29—the median, as conventionally taken, is the average (12) of the middle two values (11 and 13). (3:101)

9. **D.** The variation within a series of observations is best summarized by calculation of the standard deviation, which is a measure of the scatter of the observations around their mean. A large standard deviation shows that there is a wide scatter of observations around the mean value, while a small standard deviation shows that the observations are concentrated around the mean with little variation between one observation and another. (3:101)

10. **C.** Ninety-five percent of individual weights fall between 140 and 200 lbs. (26:21)

11. **C.** The fiftieth percentile, by definition, is exactly in the center of any ordered distribution. This is also the definition of the median. The mean and mode would also be the fiftieth percentile only if the distribution were symmetrical. (54:82)

12. **C.** The probability for throwing a 2 would be 1:6 and the probability for throwing a 5 would be 1:6. The probability for throwing a 2 or a 5 in any throw would be 2:6 or 1:3. If events A and B (throwing a 2 or 5) are mutually exclusive—that is, if one occurs, then the other cannot possibly occur at the same time—then the probability of getting either A or B is equal to the probability of A plus the probability of B. (54:109)

13. **A.** The probability of getting a 1 in the first roll is 1:6, for getting a 2 on the second roll it is 1:6, and for getting a 5 on the last roll it is 1:6 also. Applying the multiplication rule, the probability for this particular order is $1:6 \times 1:6 \times 1:6 = 1:216$. Independence of events can be recognized by the nature of the event. Each event or roll is separate and not dependent on the outcome of a previous roll. (54:118)

14. **C.** When two things are independent, the chance that both will happen can be found by multiplying the chances (0.006 × 0.02 = 0.00012). However, it is not legitimate to multiply the chances of dependent outcomes. (18:214)

15. **E.** The expectation of life, which is derived from the life table, is a very well known mortality function; but, since it measures past not future mortality experience, it has no real prognostic significance and is not quite the simple statistic it is popularly thought to be. (23:18)

16. **E.** Throughout their lives females fare better than males. (23:19)

17. **D.** Diseases of the heart and blood vessels constitute the leading cause of death and disabling illness in the United States. They are responsible for approximately 50% of all deaths at the present time. In 1900, they accounted for only 20% of deaths. This increase is primarily due to the increasing percentage of older persons in the population. As a matter of fact, if statistical allowance is made for this change in age distribution, it is found that the death rate from this group of causes has declined since 1930, particularly in persons under the age of 45 years. Similar progress has not been made in connection with arteriosclerosis and hypertension, which are particularly common as age advances. (20:63)

18. **E.** The five leading causes of deaths among children one to four years of age in the United States are: (1) accidents, (2) congenital malformations, (3) influenza and pneumonia, (4) malignant neoplasms, (5) meningitis (except meningococcal and tuberculous). (22:328)

19. **E.** The death rate in this group has dropped from about 4 per 1,000 in 1900 to 0.6 per 1,000 at the current time. This reduction is largely attributable to success in prevention and treatment of acute communicable diseases of childhood. In addition, the lowering of the threat of tuberculosis is noteworthy. At the beginning of this century more than 36 school children per 100,000 died each year from this single cause. At the present time it is relatively inconsequential as a cause of death in this age group. (22:480)

20. **B.** The age curve of mortality has general features in common throughout the world, with variations depending chiefly on environmental factors. Mortality is high during the first year of life (infancy), drops to its lowest level in childhood, and then gradually begins to climb during the third and fourth decades. After the age of 35 or 40, the increase in mortality with age tends to be logarithmic for the remainder of the life span. (37:21)

21. **A.** There are in the United States approximately 18 million children between the ages of one and five years, customarily referred to as the preschool period. At the current time the risk of death between the first and fifth birthday is only about 1 per 1,000. This was not always the case. At the beginning of the century the death rate of this age group was about 20 per 1,000. The preschool period benefited most from many of the greatest triumphs of preventive medicine and public health. The dramatic decreases in deaths, illnesses, and disabilities in this group may be credited chiefly to the successful treatment and, what is of greater importance, to the prevention of the so-called acute communicable diseases of childhood. Improvements in mortality during this century, though touching all ages, have inevitably been much greater among the young than the old. (37:21)

22. **B.** The kitchen is the locale of the highest percentage of all home accidents (26%). The bedroom is the most fatal place, accounting for 40% of all accidental deaths in the home. This is attributable to the many toxic drugs kept there and to the dangerous habit of smoking in bed. By type of home accident, falls are the most frequent cause of death, accounting for 40% of accidental deaths. (20:588)

23. **D.** For most diseases, variation in frequency with age is greater than that with any other descriptive variable. In fact, variation with age is so commonplace that knowledge of the relationship between age and disease risk is more often useful for clarifying the effects of other variables than for its place in formulating and selecting hypotheses per se. Knowledge of age associations may, however, be very useful for administrative purposes. (12:60)

24. **A.** Because it is such a prominent aspect of infectious disease occurrence, seasonal variation has received a great deal of attention from epidemiologists. In some infectious diseases, e.g., Rocky Mountain spotted fever and equine encephalitis, seasonal variation occurs because of the seasonal character of the life cycle of the arthropod vector. In many other infectious diseases, the basis for seasonal variation remains unknown. For example, seasonal variation is one of the most striking features of poliomyelitis, a disease about which a great deal is known, and yet this feature remains unexplained. Lead poisoning, rickets, accidents, and gastric perforation are other disorders exhibiting seasonal variation. Seasonal patterns are not prominent aspects of the incidence of chronic diseases, although they may be seen with respect to severity of symptoms, as in arthritis and chronic bronchitis. (12:68)

25. **B.** No suitable tests are available for the early

detection of rheumatoid arthritis. There is some general agreement among the critics of these programs, as well as among some of the supporters, that a thorough evaluation of any screening program, including multiphasic screening, requires adequate and rigorously controlled studies in a variety of population groups. (37:1142)

26. **D.** Prophylactic silver nitrate in the eyes of newborn infants has almost eliminated ophthalmia neonatorum due to gonorrhea. Blindness resulting from congenital syphilis has been prevented by thorough treatment of pregnant women found to be infected. Retrolental fibroplasia, which occurred particularly in premature babies given high concentrations of oxygen, now rarely occurs, as its cause has been discovered. Routine tonometry in persons over 40 years of age is an important preventive measure. Cataracts occur most commonly in middle or old age and are the most common cause of blindness in the United States. (20:78)

27. **E.** Blindness in association with prematurity was first observed in the late 1930s. The disease was usually not present at birth but developed between the ages of one and six months. In infants weighing between two and three pounds, the incidence of the disease reached as high as 26%. The association between prematurity and blindness was first noticed by Terry in 1942. A concerted program of investigation ultimately disclosed the principal factor in the occurrence of this disease: overuse of oxygen in premature nurseries. (37:1263)

28. **D.** Age-adjusted death rates for coronary heart disease are highest in the United States and unusually low in Italy, Spain, Portugal, and Japan. The last-named country, peculiarly, records exceptionally high frequencies of hypertension and cerebrovascular accidents. (17:210)

29. **D.** High blood pressure is probably the most common single factor in the development of coronary heart disease. (25:162)

30. **A.** The leading cause is glomerulonephritis (56%). (37:1229)

31. **D.** In the United States about 66% of all urinary stones are composed of calcium oxalate alone or mixed with calcium phosphate. About 15% are composed of magnesium ammonium phosphate. Uric acid and cystine stones make up about 10%. The remainder consist of stones made up of xanthine, silicates, or a protein matrix. (37:1237)

32. **E.** Wilson's disease, a herditary copper storage illness, has not been described as a result of chronic industrial exposure to copper. (21:57)

33. **E.** The pathognomonic sign of Wilson's disease is the Kayser-Fleischer ring. Large quantities of copper are excreted in the urine and deposited in the tissues. Oral penicillamine is the drug of choice. (21:57)

34. **A.** While accurate data on the number of children suffering from various handicapping conditions are difficult to secure, the following rough estimates of prevalence of certain handicaps among children below 21 years of age may serve to indicate how frequent these conditions are (prevalence per 100 children): emotional problems 10, mental retardation 3, orthopedic problems 2, speech defects 2, cardiac defects 1. (20:158)

35. **B.** Among patients hospitalized for mental illness, schizophrenia is the most common condition, accounting for 45.6% of the total. The frequencies of other important conditions are mental disease of the senium 12.2%, manic depression 7.6%, syphilitic psychosis 6.7%, and psychosis with mental deficiency 6%. Alcoholic and involutional psychoses each account for about 3% of those hospitalized. (22:514)

36. **B.** Among professionals, those in medicine, and especially psychiatrists and psychoanalysts, have the highest rate. Indeed, the annual suicide rate among physicians in the United States is at least 33 per 100,000—three times the national average. Among psychiatrists and psychoanalysts the rate is 70 per 100,000 per year. The rates among the military are highest during peacetime, but rates for the military and most other groups drop sharply when a nation is confronted with a military emergency. (22:526)

37. **E.** Congenital thyroid deficiency is the most important metabolic disease currently recognized by infant screening. Galactosemia results from deficiency of the enzyme galactokinase. Removal of galactose-containing foods from the diet, especially milk, leads to a dramatic improvement in the patient, and all clinical features except mental retardation may improve or disappear. Maple syrup urine disease, so named because of the characteristic odor of urine and perspiration, is a disorder of branched-chain amino acids. Treatment is based on a diet that limits the corresponding amino acids. Homocysteinuria is caused by the diminishing activity of cystachioline synthetase, an enzyme important in the pathway that converts methionine to cysteine. (37:1260)

38. **B.** Although many patients have symptoms early in life, the diagnosis is rarely made before the age of 21. One of the most intriguing epidemiologic features of multiple sclerosis is its geographic distribution. The disease has been shown to be rare between the equator and latitudes 30 to 35 degrees and to become more common with increasing latitude thereafter. This relationship is clearly demonstrated for the Northern Hemisphere in both morbidity and mortality. (12:266)

39. **D.** An intravenous dose of Tensilon produces a brief remission of symptoms if they are caused by an exacerbation of the illness but further weakens patients suffering from an overdose of medication. (2:282)

40. **D.** The addict frequently does not know how much he is actually taking. As a result, serious toxic reactions and even death may occur from an overdose. Overdose is estimated to kill 1% of New York's addicts each year. (22:558)

41. **E.** If the present rates continue, about one third of the population of the United States will develop cancer at some time in their lives and about one fifth will die of the disease. There are more than 600,000 new cases of cancer (exclusive of carcinoma in situ and basal and squamous cell carcinomas of the skin) and over 350,000 deaths attributed to the disease annually in this country alone. (12:451)

42. **A.** Well over 80% of all cancers are believed to result primarily from environmental factors. (48:136)

43. **B.** Cancer of the respiratory tract causes about 80,000 deaths in the United States each year; 94% of these are due to cancer of the trachea, bronchus, and lung. As in many other countries, death rates for respiratory cancer have been increasing in both men and women. In women, a marked increase in age-specific rates took place starting in about 1955, but the rates are still about four times as high in men as in women. The increase during the past 20 years has been somewhat grater in nonwhites than in whites. There is considerable variation within the United States in respiratory cancer mortality rates. These have been most often presented for lung cancer, for which maps by county have been published. These geographic patterns have suggested hypotheses about etiology. Significant occupational exposures or hazardous emissions from certain industries have sometimes been identified in this way. (37:1252)

44. **C.** The religious ritual of circumcision appears to play a role in cancer prevention. This ritual is thought by many to be the reason for the low incidence of not only cancer of the glans penis among Jewish men but also cancer of the cervix among Jewish women. (48:537)

45. **D.** To date, Japanese migrants have not displayed a tendency for their originally low rates of breast cancer to rise to the level of that in the United States. The incidence of breast cancer has increased in most western countries, though in the United States this increase has been more apparent for non-whites than whites. Other factors that have at one time or another been associated with a higher risk of female breast cancer are: ethnic group (Jewish), marital status (single), race (caucasian), age at first pregnancy (older), number of pregnancies (fewer), age at menarche (earlier), history of benign breast disease, socioeconomic status (higher), nulliparity, high-dose radiation exposure, a family history of breast cancer. (24:520)

46. **C.** The Food and Drug Administration (FDA) regulates the exclusion of cancer-causing substances from food. (50:158)

47. **E.** If the current rate of increase (1.9% compounded annually) continues, by the year 2050 the world's population will reach an almost incomprehensive 15 billion, and this is less than 70 years in the future. (22:74)

48. **D.** In terms of population, an increase of 200,000 per day is equivalent to adding a city the size of St. Petersburg each day or the total combined populations of the United Kingdom and the Scandinavian countries each year. (22:75)

49. **E.** Year 1975: Latin America 2.7%, Africa 2.6%, Asia 2.1%, North America 0.9%, Europe 0.6%, world 1.9%. (22:75)

50. **E.** In the United States the decennial census was established in 1790, enumerating some four million persons along the eastern seaboard, and has continued in unbroken sequence since that date. The last was carried out in 1980. Population estimates are made for intercensus years. Plans are in preparation to run censuses in the United States every five years. (17:111)

51. **C.** The increase or decrease in world population is the difference between the number of live births and the number of deaths. The rate of growth is commonly expressed as the difference between the crude birth and crude death rates. Migration may be a factor in rates of growth within a country or region but does not directly affect world rates of growth. A useful formula to determine the number of years required for a population to double at a specified annual rate of increase is: years to double = 70 ÷ annual rate of increase (%). (8:471)

52. **A.** A useful formula to determine the annual rate of increase required to double the population is: Rate of increase (%) = 70 ÷ number of years to double the population. (8:471)

53. **A.** Hormonal contraception (oral contraceptives) has become one of the most widely used methods of fertility control in many western countries during the past decade. Its acceptability in these areas is due to the esthetics of not needing to employ a device or agent immediately associated with the sexual act and the negligible failure rate when properly

followed. Intrauterine devices have proved relatively safe. Excessive bleeding and pelvic inflammation have been the most frequent complications. The failure rate is much lower than that of traditional contraceptive measures. Vaginal foam tablets have high failure rates but they may be desirable to furnish one of the most reliable nonclinical agents to women who want to take the contraceptive responsibility. One of the first steps in any family planning program should be to ensure that condoms are widely available at low cost. This method, even when correctly practiced, has had high failure rates. Its acceptability to some families may at least contribute to their acceptance of the concept of family planning. (23:545)

54. **B.** Respiratory ailments are by far the commonest cause of sickness (absenteeism), followed by disorders of the digestive system. (20:237)

55. **C.** Currently, approximately six work days per person per year are lost as a result of illness or injury. (20:237)

56. **B.** In general, any licensed physician is considered to qualify as an expert witness in controversies dealing with medical questions. Specialization is not necessary, and the expert witness may give an opinion even if he never before saw either litigant and even if he never before observed a similar case. (22:195)

57. **A.** The largest single item of expenditure, representing more than 40% of the total personal health care dollar, was for hospital care, including both inpatient and outpatient service. Physician services are the next largest type of expenditure, amounting to almost 19% of total. (8:548)

58. **B.** Approximately two thirds of all infant deaths occur during the first month; about one third occur on the first day of life. (20:146)

59. **A.** Between 1960 and 1965, the infant mortality rate decreased only 5% but it dropped 19% between 1965 and 1970. The rate for 1977 was 14.1 per thousand live births. Considerable disparity exists between the rate for white (about 12) and that for black (about 22) infants. In general, the highest rates are in the lowest socioeconomic groups, both white and nonwhite. (20:146)

60. **E.** Approximately 8.8% of all births in the United States are premature. Among white infants in the United States and Canada, the frequency of low birth weight ranges from 5 to 8%. Among nonwhite infants it is as high as 12%. (20:153)

61. **E.** The place of delivery is important in making any assessment of the status of maternity care in a community. A high proportion of hospital deliveries usually indicates superior services. The trends in many countries have been steadily toward an even larger percentage of deliveries in hospitals. The proportion of births occurring at home has declined steadily in the United States for the past 50 years, so that home births constitute in most states less than 1% of the total. Recently, however, some areas have recorded an increase in the number of home births. (37:1781)

62. **A.** Among newborn white infants, the proportion of twins is therefore approximately 2%, since each twin confinement yields two infants. In such estimates the substantial ethnic and geographic variation in rates of twinning must be considered. (33:316)

63. **D.** Some diseases are due exclusively to genetic factors: Examples are hemophilia, fibrocystic disease of the pancreas, multiple polyposis of the colon, sickle cell anemia. In other diseases, genetic factors appear to exert an important influence. Examples of this group include deaf mutism, cataracts, and parkinsonism. There are many diseases in which genetic factors appear to exercise some influence, although the exact extent to which this is important is not known. Examples include cancer of the breast, gout, diabetes, epilepsy, and asthma. There are many other diseases that do not appear to be related in any way to genetic factors, such as measles and pneumonia. (20:158)

64. **C.** This is a very crude measure of risk because of the great variation with age; it is useful as a measure of population decrement due to natural causes. (50:61)

65. **D.** Prevalence rate determined from cross-sectional studies. (50:61)

66. **E.** Approaches a measure of risk, especially if also specific for sex. (50:61)

67. **A.** Also called "crude cause of death rate" because age is not specified. (50:61)

68. **D.** The prevalence rate measures numbers of existing diseases in a population. (50:29)

69. **E.** Definition of neonatal mortality. (23:22)

70. **B.** Definition of early neonatal mortality. (23:22)

71. **D.** Definition of late neonatal mortality. (23:22)

72. **C.** Definition of postneonatal mortality. (23:22)

73. **A.** Definition of perinatal mortality. (23:22)

74. **E.** The denominator might be the total number of women who became pregnant during the year. This

is a difficult or impossible number to obtain, so another figure is employed—that of the number of live births occurring in the population during the year. Stillbirths are not included, as the stillbirth data are so unreliable. (8:135)

75. **E.** The denominator of the cause-specific death rate is the estimated mid-interval population. Cause-specific death rates indicate the probability of death or illness owing to a specific disease or condition. They are useful in the study of trends and comparisons of health status between populations, since different patterns of mortality and morbidity commonly reflect variation of lifestyle and socioeconomic development. (12:41)

76. **D.** The denominator of the age-specific death rate is the average population in the same age group during the same period. (8:136)

77. **A.** The denominator of the crude death rate is the estimated midyear population. Crude death rates are particularly misleading for conditions that are heavily weighted at the extremes of life. They are usually expressed as the number of deaths registered during a given period of time per 1,000 population. (8:135)

78. **E.** This description corresponds to the "infant mortality rate." (8:136)

79. **A.** $1 + 7 = 8; 8 \div 2 = 4$. (54:368)

80. **B.** $7 - 1 = 6$. (54:368)

81. **B.** $(1 - 3 - 4 - 5 - \underline{6} - 6 - 6 - 7 - 7)$. (54:368)

82. **B.** The number 6 is repeated three times. (54:368)

83. **C.** Sum of quantities (45) divided by the number of quantities (9) = 5. (54:367)

84. **D.** The median is that score in an ordered distribution above which and below which half the frequencies fall. It is the middle score in an ordered set of scores. (58:55)

85. **C.** The arithmetic mean is the sum of the quantities divided by the number of quantities. Sometimes the mean is referred to as the "average." (58:55)

86. **B.** The mode (or modal value) is the score or value that occurs most often in a set of data. It is the maximum point on the frequency distribution curve. (58:55)

87. **A.** The range is simply a statement of the difference between the smallest and largest scores in a distribution. In some instances the range is expressed as "high minus low, plus 1." (54:77)

88. **E.** The midrange is the arithmetic mean of the largest and smallest values in a set of observations. (54:77)

89. **D.** Included between $+1$ and -1 standard deviation (68.26%). (26:21)

90. **A.** Included between $+3$ and -3 standard deviation (99.72%). (26:21)

91. **B.** Included between $+2$ and -2 standard deviation (95.44%). (26:21)

92. **A.** Age group one to four: accidents. (37:1135)

93. **A.** Age group five to 14: accidents. (37:1135)

94. **A.** Age group 15–24: accidents. (37:1135)

95. **A.** Age group 25–44: accidents. (37:1135)

96. **C.** Age group 45–64: diseases of the heart. (37:1135)

97. **E.** Amphetamines. (22:556)

98. **D.** Heroin. (22:556)

99. **C.** LSD. (22:556)

100. **B.** Codeine. (22:556)

101. **A.** Barbiturates. (22:556)

102. **C.** The highest incidence of skin cancer is found in eastern Australia, where Caucasians lacking the pigmented skin that protects dark-skinned races tend to expose themselves excessively in sport and work. (48:136)

103. **A.** The concoction is the Asian equivalent of chewing gum. Cancer of the mouth is rare in the United States. (48:137)

104. **B.** Substantial evidence now exists that one causative factor in nasopharyngeal cancer may be the Epstein-Barr virus. (48:137)

105. **E.** Different factors, possibly a combination of many, may be responsible in different areas of cancer of the esophagus. (48:137)

106. **D.** Those with pernicious anemia have a four to five times greater risk of developing gastric cancer. (48:138)

107. **D.** Cancers of the colon and rectum, believed to be related to diet, were found in both sexes at above average rates in the Northeast United States and in urban areas along the Great Lakes. Surprisingly, breast cancer showed a similar pattern, suggesting that this disease may have an environmental factor in common with cancers of the large intestine. (36:X)

108. **C.** Scientists have known for many years that sunlight is a major cause of skin cancer and that darker-skinned persons are less susceptible. (36:X)

109. **E.** The incidence of stomach cancer in those countries is also higher than the United States average. (36:X)

110. **B.** Of the 21 counties in New Jersey, 18 have bladder cancer rates in the highest decile of male rates for all U.S. counties. In Salem County, New Jersey, the rate is 16.1 × 100,000 population. (36:X)

111. **A.** The Bantu of Johannesburg, South Africa, have an over-all cancer incidence rate about half that of the U.S. white population, and yet they have rates of esophageal, liver, and cervical cancer that are much higher than those in the United States. (12:454)

112. **B.** Primary liver cancer is uncommon in western countries. It is associated with both a toxin (aflatoxin) produced by a fungus *(Aspergillus flavus)* growing on crops stored in moist, warm conditions, and also with infection caused by the virus hepatitis B. Improved methods of food storage could reduce the growth of *Aspergillus flavus*. (48:140)

113. **A.** In terms of geographical distribution, polyps—nonmalignant tumors of the bowel—are rare where cancer is rare and exceedingly common where cancer is common. (48:139)

114. **C.** The evidence is strongly suggestive that infestation with *Schistosoma haematobium* increases the risk of developing bladder cancer. (37:1161)

115. **E.** Excess of biliary carcinoma is generally attributed to the high rate of cholelithiasis. (48:227)

116. **D.** Women with Plummer-Vinson syndrome are reportedly at high risk of oral cancer. (37:1459)

117. **C.** Osteosarcoma occurred among workers painting watch dials with luminous paint. "Tipping" their brushes with tongue or lip to obtain a fine point, they swallowed considerable amounts of radium. (12:461)

118. **A.** Benzene has been clearly shown to be leukemogenic at exposure levels that have characterized a variety of industries in the past. (12:461)

119. **B.** Angiosarcoma of the liver is a rare tumor, with only about 20 cases occurring annually in the United States. Previously known causes were thorotrast and heavy exposure to arsenic trioxide in insecticides. The causal agent is the vinyl chloride monomer. (12:461)

120. **D.** Various environmental factors have already been implicated as causal agents for different forms of cancer. This concept had its origin in Percival Pott's report of the increased risk of scrotal cancer among English chimney sweeps in 1775. (37:1152)

121. **E.** There is an increased incidence of nasal cavity and nasal sinuses cancer among workers exposed to wood dust. (37:1157)

122. **D.** Studies of radiologists leave no doubt that persons receiving high doses of radiation are at substantially increased risk of leukemia. (12:460)

123. **C.** Patients with xeroderma pigmentosum show extreme sensitivity to sunlight and tend to develop skin cancer with exposure to sun. (50:24)

124. **B.** The evidence is convincing that the tumors in the alpha-naphthylamine workers were actually due to contamination with beta isomers. Aniline itself is no longer believed to be carcinogenic. (21:259)

125. **A.** The risk of lung cancer in nickel refining disappeared when the process was altered in the 1920s and arsenic-free sulphuric acid was used to remove copper from the ore. (61:103)

126. **A.** Certain occupational exposures increase the risk of lung cancer—chromate production is one of them. (61:103)

127. **D.** There is an increased risk of vaginal carcinoma among young women born of mothers who were treated during pregnancy with synthetic estrogen (diethylstilbestrol) to prevent abortion. (12:462)

128. **E.** The high incidence of leukemia has been related to chloramphenicol therapy. (50:132)

129. **E.** Therapeutic radiation for ankylosing spondilitis has been associated with a high incidence of leukemia. (50:133)

130. **E.** Cytoxan (for rheumatoid arthritis) has been associated with a high incidence of leukemia. (50:133)

131. **B.** Cancer of the thyroid, thyroid adenomas, and other tumors of the head and neck have occurred with excessive frequency in children treated with x-ray for enlargement of the thymus in infancy. The risk is dose-related, compatible with a linear relationship. (12:461)

132. **B.** Fluoroscopic examination of the chest has been followed by a higher-than-expected number of cases of breast cancer. (39:57)

133. **A.** Angiosarcoma of the liver and leukemia have occurred following the use in the 1940s of thorotrast, a radioactive contrast medium containing thorium. (12:461)

134. **C.** Evidence suggests that herpes simplex virus of the genital tract (HSV-2) is etiologically implicated in cancer of the cervix. (37:1161)

135. **D.** Scrotal and other skin cancers were reported among British cotton mule spinners prior to 1953. (21:210)

136. **E.** Mesothelioma has been reported among "pipe fitters" exposed to asbestos. (21:351)

137. **D.** One of the strongest associations of disease with birth order is that of hypertrophic pyloric stenosis, a disease with onset usually within six weeks of birth. First births experience a rate three times as high as that of births after the third. (33:326)

138. **A.** The incidence of Down's syndrome is less than one per 1,000 in infants born to mothers under 30 years of age but more than one per 100 in infants of mothers over 40. (33:327)

139. **D.** The effect of previous pregnancies, through changes in the maternal antibody system, is seen in the increase in frequency and severity of erythroblastosis with increasing birth order. (33:324)

140. **A.** Another striking association with maternal age occurs with the frequency of dizygotic twinning, which is about six times higher for the maternal age group 35–39 years than for the age groups 15–19. Associations with the age of the father seem less frequent. (33:327)

141. **D.** The more prolonged and difficult labor characteristic of first pregnancies may lead to higher rates of abnormalities resulting from anoxia, trauma, prolonged anesthesia, and other factors related to the confinement. An intriguing suggestion in this connection is that the relatively high frequency of patent ductus arteriosus in first births may be due in part to such factors acting at a time when the physiologic stimulus for closure should occur. (33:325)

142. **D.** Sulfasalazine should be given cautiously during pregnancy; the potential teratogenicity has not been fully investigated. Kernicterus may occur in newborn infants. (2:971)

143. **A.** High blood levels of chloramphenicol in premature and full-term infants frequently cause a toxic reaction referred to as the Grey syndrome. (2:1252)

144. **E.** Administration of streptomycin sulfate to pregnant women has been reported to diminish eighth cranial nerve function in the fetus. (2:1292)

145. **B.** Tetracyclines should be avoided during pregnancy because they are attracted to embryonic and growing osseous tissue. Temporary depression of bone growth occurs in the fetus and young children. (2:1270)

146. **C.** Magnesium sulfate is generally safe but may suppress skeletal muscle activity in the neonate. (2:798)

147. **B.** Androgens and anabolic steroids are usually contraindicated in pregnant women because of possible masculinization of female fetuses. (2:657)

148. **E.** Orally administered anticoagulants cross the placenta and have been associated with birth defects. Anticoagulants should be discontinued after the thirty-seventh week since there is a risk of hemorrhage in the fetus, particularly during labor. (2:1077)

149. **A.** Cleft lip has been associated with the use of diazepam during the first trimester of pregnancy. Intravenous administration of more than 30 mg of diazepam during the final 15 hours of labor can produce the floppy infant syndrome. (2:148)

150. **C.** An infant born to a mother who abuses amphetamines may be agitated and have hyperglycemia at birth. (2:219)

151. **D.** Excessive amounts of vitamin D during pregnancy are potentially dangerous to the fetus (they may cause supravalvular aortic stenosis, vascular injury, and suppression of parathyroid function with resultant hypocalcemic tetany in the neonate. (2:824)

152. **A.** With phenobarbital use a hemorrhagic diathesis has been observed occasionally. (2:151)

153. **E.** Since propylthiouracil crosses the placenta, goiter and hypothyroidism may occur in the neonate. (2:771)

154. **D.** When given parenterally for treating eclampsia, reserpine passes through the placental circulation and may cause drowsiness, nasal congestion, cyanosis, and anorexia in the newborn infant. (2:569)

155. **C.** If used in excessive quantities, particularly in paracervical block, local anesthetics may accumulate and cause fetal bradycardia, expulsion of meconium before birth, and marked central nervous system depression after birth. (2:291)

156. **B.** The use of antipsychotic drugs during pregnancy probably should be restricted to psychotic patients who require continued medication. Phenothiazines cross the placenta and prolonged extrapyramidal effects may appear in the infant. (2:171)

157. **A.** Incidence (attack, case) rates allow for an individual being counted more than once as a case if the condition is one for which this is possible (e.g., accidents, colds). (37:16)

158. **B.** Prevalence determinations are useful for measuring the frequency in a population of states that are either permanent or of considerable duration; thus they are of value in chronic disease. (37:16)

159. **B.** The prevalence rate equals the number of existing cases of disease divided by the population at risk at the time of measurement. The prevalence rate is, therefore, a static measure of disease frequency. (12:39)

160. **A.** Incidence rates are useful for studying disease causation and the evaluation of preventive measures. (12:40)

161. **B.** A birth rate is an incidence rate. However, a birth defect rate is a prevalence rate. (39:29)

162. **A.** Sensitivity is the ability to identify correctly those who have the disease. Specificity is the ability to identify correctly those who do not have the disease. (47:56)

163. **B.** The number of true negatives divided by the total number of persons without the disease represents the specificity of the association between not having the disease and not having the symptom. (50:105)

164. **A.** Sensitivity, one of the two components of the validity of a test, is defined as the characteristic of a test, sign, or symptom that estimates the strength of the association of the test result with the presence of the disease. It is simply the proportion of the diseased who have the symptom. (50:105)

165. **B.** Specificity, one of the two components of the validity of a test, is defined as the characteristic of a test, sign, or symptom that estimates the uniqueness of the association of the test result with the presence of the disease. (50:105)

166. **C.** In actuality, values of 100% seldom, if ever, occur for either sensitivity or specificity. (50:83)

167. **C.** The purpose of retrospective and prospective studies is to identify the presence of an association between a risk factor and disease. (50:91)

168. **A.** The "negative predictive value of a negative association" and the "positive predictive value of a positive association" are corresponding terms for prospective associations. (50:84)

169. **B.** "Sensitivity" and "specificity" refer to retrospective associations. (50:84)

170. **A.** The cost of a prospective study is relatively expensive; the cost of a retrospective study is relatively inexpensive. (50:96)

171. **B.** Retrospective analyis relates events in an "after-before" sequence, in contrast to prospective analysis, which addresses associations in a "before-after" manner with respect to cause. (50:83)

172. **A.** Validity is synonymous with accuracy. In screening programs the validity of a screening test is evaluated by the sensitivity and specificity of the test. (50:106)

173. **B.** If repeated measuring of some variable continues to give the same results, the measure is reliable. (54:134)

174. **B.** Reliability is synonymous with precision. (50:105)

175. **A.** Validity is how well a measure does what it says it does. (50:134)

176. **C.** Validity and reliability are two characteristics of measurement. (50:134)

177. **A.** A triangular broad-based pattern reflects high birth and high death rates over a long period of time and is characteristic of the so-called "developing countries." (50:61)

178. **A.** High maternal mortality rates are associated with developing countries. Poor socioeconomic conditions and cultural factors often are associated with unfavorable areas. (8:138)

179. **A.** The population growth rates may exceed 3.5% per year in developing countries. (8:471)

180. **B.** Life expectancy and the median age of the population are both high in economically developed countries. (50:61)

181. **B.** In wealthy nations overnutrition makes obesity a common problem and is associated with a high prevalence of coronary heart disease, diabetes, dental caries, and numerous other conditions. (37:6)

182. **C.** (37:1349)

183. **A.** (37:1349)

184. **D.** (37:1349)

185. **D.** (37:1349)

186. **D.** (37:1349)

187. **E.** Among white males in the United States suicide death rates increase consistently with each age group, from 9.3 per 100,000 males between 15 and 24 years to 65.1 per 100,000 in those 85 years and older. Among white females rates peak at 12.5 per 100,000 among those 45 to 54 years, then decrease. (22:525)

188. **A.** Alcoholism affects predominantly men in the ratio of 3 or more to 1, although the gap is constantly closing. It is significantly greater in urban areas. Alcoholics lose more work time than nonalcoholics but they do not appear to suffer a higher rate of occupational accidents. (22:539)

189. **E.** Withdrawal syndromes following prolonged exposure to agents that have toxic effects on the central nervous system also occur. The best known of these follows a period of many days of heavy alcohol ingestion and is known as delirium tremens. (37:1329)

190. **E.** There can be no doubt that the main cause of lung cancer is cigarette smoking. The risk of dying of lung cancer is between 8 and 15 times higher among cigarette smokers than among nonsmokers. Certain occupational exposures, such as involved in radioactive ore mining, coke oven work, and smelting and refining copper, lead, and zinc ores, are well-established occupational risks. (37:1253)

191. **E.** Lung cancer is an occupational disease among asbestos workers. It occurs much more frequently in asbestos workers than in the general population. Other cancers are also asbestos-related, including cancer of the stomach and the nose and throat. There is also a related very rare form of cancer, occurring in the outer lining of the lung and other membranes, called mesothelioma. (50:3)

192. **A.** Lower socioeconomic status, early frequent sexual activity, and multiple pregnancies have been found to be associated with elevated rates of cervical cancer in various ethnic groups. There is no substantial evidence of a genetic predisposition to carcinoma of the cervix. (48:227)

193. **E.** The disease is uncommon under the age of two or over 16 years. The lymphoma is considered a manifestation of the Epstein-Barr (EB) virus infection acting against a background of immunosuppression caused by endemic malaria. Chemotherapy: methotrexate, nitrogen mustard, cyclophosphamide. (35:12)

194. **A.** For only three cancer sites—gallbladder, thyroid gland, and breast—is the mortality higher among women than men. (29:95)

195. **E.** These four types of cancer are closely associated epidemiologically with a number of other diseases characteristic of economically developed communities and collectively referred to as "western diseases." (48:140)

196. **E.** Address inquiries to the American Board of Preventive Medicine, Secretary-Treasurer, Graduate School of Public Health, University of Pittsburgh, Pittsburgh, Pennsylvania 15261, U.S.A.

197. **E.** Early recognition of multiple pregnancy makes possible more intensive prenatal care and, therefore, can contribute to the prevention of prematurity. Similarly, early effective prenatal care may reduce toxemia, while birth-control measures may be indicated in the presence of chronic hypertension in a woman. (12:153)

198. **E.** Infectious agents such as the etiologic agents of syphilis, rubella, and toxoplasmosis have been implicated in the genesis of congenital malformations. Chemicals implicated are those such as thalidomide. Physical agents are those such as ionic radiation, x-rays, and radium. Injury of the uterine contents by trauma may produce death or anomalies of the embryo. Blows to the abdomen, automobile accidents, or falls are not uncommon and may result in congenital malformations. (8:169)

199. **A.** The crude birth rate is a good measure of the

overall effect of fertility on the current growth rate of a population. However, it does not measure the risk of childbearing. (37:1505)

200. **A.** The denominator is the specified population at the midpoint of the time period. (26:117)

201. **D.** This rate is calculated on the basis of live births. It should be recognized that, in multiple pregnancies, each live-born child is included in the denominator, but only one woman is exposed to the risk of dying. This inclusion of multiple births in the denominator does not compensate for the omission of pregnancies resulting in other than live births. (26:118)

202. **B.** The basic characteristic of incidence-type rates is that time is part of the units: cases/population/time. Prevalence-type rates are simply cases per population; a cure rate may be persons cured/100 persons tested. (39:67)

203. **E.** As customarily used, the term attack rate describes the incidence of disease when the population at risk is exposed for a short period of time, as in an acute epidemic. (39:29)

204. **A.** Central tendency measures are descriptive statistics that are used to summarize a group's performance in terms of where the scores tend to be concentrated. Three central tendency measures are commonly used—the mean, the median, or the mode, depending on the circumstances. The range is a measure of dispersion. (54:366)

205. **E.** By dispersion we mean a measure that indicates the extent to which a set of scores deviate from, or disperse themselves around, some measure of central tendency for that set. Range, percentiles, semi-interquartile range, and standard deviation are measures of dispersion. (54:78)

206. **E.** The advantages of the standard deviation are that it uses every observation and it is mathematically manageable. The disadvantage is that it is very sensitive to outliers. (44:18)

207. **E.** Percentiles are frequently encountered in literature in applied fields. Percentiles divide the total range into 100 parts, each of which has the same number of cases. Deciles divide the total range into ten parts, each of which contain ten percentiles. (28:14)

208. **B.** Quartiles are the percentiles that divide the distribution into quarters—the 25th, 50th and 75th percentiles are in the first, second, and third quartiles. (54:87)

209. **A.** If the value of a variable changes, by whole numbers—for example, counts of children in a family—the variable is known as discrete. (3:98)

210. **A.** A variable is continuous if, conceptually, it could take on any value in certain intervals. Continuous scales are used for measurements when fractions are real and meaningful, such as 12.1 gm hemoglobin per 100 ml, or 5.3 mg uric acid. (26:6)

211. **E.** In statistics, the term "population" has a slightly different meaning from the one given to it in ordinary speech. (56:16)

212. **A.** Random sampling is a procedure for selecting individuals (or any other unit) from a population such that each individual has an equal or known chance of appearing in the sample. The basic problem is to find a sampling method that gives the investigator and his readers insurance that personal bias, conscious or unconscious, did not enter into the selection. (17:168)

213. **A.** A negative (−) sign denotes that an upward movement of one characteristic is accompanied by a downward movement of the other. The correlation coefficient ranges from −1, when all the points lie on a line that slopes down, to +1, when all the points lie on a line that slopes up. (18:135)

214. **A.** Adding the same number to all the values of one variable, or multiplying all the values of one variable by the same positive number, will not change the correlation coefficient. (18:127)

215. **E.** At the beginning of the century 61% of deaths were caused by infectious and parasitic diseases and only 28% by chronic and metabolic diseases. The situation is now reversed, with over 80% of deaths caused by chronic and metabolic disease and less than 1% by infectious or parasitic diseases. The 12 leading causes of death in the United States are: diseases of the heart, malignant neoplasms, cerebrovascular disease, accidents, influenza and pneumonia, diseases of early infancy, diabetes mellitus, arteriosclerosis, cirrhosis of the liver, suicide, bronchitis, emphysema and asthma, and homicide. (22:11)

216. **E.** Accidents in the home are particularly important because of their frequency, which approaches one half of all accidents. In terms of severity, they account for one third of disabling injuries and, as measured by deaths per 1,000 injuries, they exceed occupational accidents. The kitchen is the locale of the highest percentage of all home accidents (26%), and the bedroom is the most fatal place, accounting for 40% of all accidental deaths in the home. This is attributable to the many toxic drugs kept there plus the dangerous habit of some people of smoking in bed. Falls are the most frequent cause of death, accounting

for 32% of accidental deaths. Fires account for 21%, poisons for 14%, suffocation for 10%, firearms for 5%, and gas for 4%. Among females the highest home injury rate is in the lowest income group, whereas among males it is just the opposite, with the home injury rate in the highest income group being twice the rate for males in the lowest income group. (22:676)

217. **C.** Duodenal ulcer and coronary heart disease occur primarily in men; cholecystitis and thyrotoxicosis are more frequent in women. (12:113)

218. **D.** Women are 50% more likely than men to have diabetes. Gout, cirrhosis, and arteriosclerotic heart disease occur more commonly in men. (12:260)

219. **D.** The prevalence of hypertension is greater among blacks at every age. In the United States, radiologic surveys indicate a prevalence in black women of approximately 40 per 100,000 persons. This may be 12 to 15 times more common than in white women. Pyloric stenosis of the pylorus occurs in the white population of the United States with a frequency of about 1.2 per 1,000 live births. The nonwhite rate is less than half that for whites. (12:205)

220. **A.** Diseases transmitted from animals to human beings, including those involving arthropod vectors, are more frequent in rural areas or the suburban outskirts of the cities. The incidence of lung cancer is nearly twice as great in urban as in rural men (age-adjusted rates). (17:234)

221. **A.** Many factors are believed to contribute to the cause of this disease. Risk factors include high intakes of fat, smoking, obesity, diabetes, and sedentary occupations. (48:146)

222. **D.** The usual ages at first admission are: schizophrenia 16-35 years; alcoholic psychosis 25-54 years; manic depressive psychosis 35-50 years; senile psychosis 60+ years. (22:515)

223. **A.** The higher a person is on the socioeconomic scale, the less the chance will be of developing a psychologic illness, except manic depressive psychosis. (22:515)

224. **A.** General paresis due to inadequate treatment of syphilis is now rare among patients admitted to mental hospitals. Pellagra has also disappeared, for practical purposes, as a cause of mental illness in the United States. Among other steps taken to prevent brain damage are adequate measures against lead poisoning and against a variety of drugs that may produce brain injury. (12:206)

225. **B.** There is no significant difference between the sexes with respect to the incidence of mental deficiency or of senile psychoses. Personality disorders are twice as frequent and alcoholic psychoses are about four or five times as frequent in men as in women. (22:516)

226. **E.** About 50% more women than men enter hospitals because of schizophrenia and manic depression. The incidence of psychoneuroses appears to be about twice as high in women as in men, whereas involutional psychoses are three times as high. (22:515)

CHAPTER TWO

Epidemiology

Directions: Each of the questions or incomplete statements below is followed by five suggested answers or completions. Select the BEST answer in each case.

1. At the World Health Assembly in May of 1980, the World Health Organization (WHO) declared the world free of

   A. plague
   B. cholera
   C. yellow fever
   D. smallpox
   E. measles

2. The leading cause of death in the world today is

   A. tuberculosis
   B. heart disease
   C. malaria
   D. accidents
   E. schistosomiasis

3. The interval between infection by an agent and maximal infectivity of the host is known as the

   A. incubation period
   B. generation time
   C. communicable period
   D. gradient of infection
   E. none of the above

4. The incubation period in human beings may be as long as six months to a year for which of the following?

   A. infectious hepatitis
   B. typhoid fever
   C. rabies
   D. poliomyelitis
   E. serum hepatitis

5. Excretion of the agent terminates before clinical recovery in which of the following?

   A. typhoid fever
   B. diphtheria
   C. mumps
   D. measles
   E. none of the above

6. Which of the following statements about Legionnaire's disease is (are) correct?

   A. a multisystem disease
   B. the attack rate is between 1 and 5% of people exposed
   C. the incubation period averages five to six days
   D. the mortality rate is approximately 15%
   E. all of the above

7. Carriers play an important role in the epidemiology of

   A. poliomyelitis
   B. meningococcal meningitis

29

C. typhoid fever
D. diphtheria
E. all of the above

8. Which of the following fails to produce a significant proportion of inapparent infections?

   A. polio
   B. mumps
   C. diphtheria
   D. pneumonia
   E. measles

9. Communicable diseases transmissible between animals and human beings (zoonoses) include all of the following *except*

   A. clonorchiasis
   B. echinococcosis
   C. poliomyelitis
   D. diphyllobothriasis
   E. fascioliasis

10. Which of the following does *not* require an insect vector to reach human beings?

    A. rabies
    B. cowpox
    C. psittacosis (ornithosis)
    D. salmonellae
    E. all of the above

11. Which of the following infections presumably results from penetration of abraded skin or mucous membrane?

    A. louse-borne typhus
    B. malaria
    C. Weil's disease
    D. typhoid fever
    E. yellow fever

12. Which of the following diseases may be transmitted by blood transfusion?

    A. cytomegalovirus disease
    B. syphilis
    C. toxoplasmosis
    D. viral hepatitis
    E. all of the above

13. Which of the following primary pathogens is responsible for the highest number of nosocomial infections?

    A. *Escherichia coli*
    B. *Staphylococcus aureus*
    C. *Klebsiella* species
    D. Group A streptococcus
    E. *Pseudomonas aeruginosa*

14. Which of the following is the most frequent site of infection in nosocomial (hospital-acquired) infections?

    A. urinary tract
    B. surgical wound
    C. lower respiratory tract
    D. skin—nonsurgical area
    E. upper respiratory tract

15. The white blood cell count may be elevated in

    A. brucellosis
    B. measles
    C. typhoid fever
    D. yellow fever
    E. none of the above

16. The risk of acquiring malaria depends on which of the following local conditions?

    A. density and habits of mosquito vectors
    B. weather
    C. altitude
    D. prevalence of infection
    E. all of the above

17. Chills and fever of a typical malaria paroxysm are initiated in which of the following stages of the parasite life cycle?

    A. as the mosquito feeds from the human bloodstream, it releases malaria sporozoites, which enter liver cells (exoerythrocytic stage)
    B. after the parasite matures, the liver cell ruptures and releases numerous merozoites
    C. the merozoites invade the red blood cells, starting the erythrocytic stage of an infection

D. within the red blood cells the parasites mature, become schizonts, and divide again into merozoites
E. the infected red blood cells rupture, and merozoites repeat the cycle by invading other red blood cells

18. Which of the following is the drug of choice for the suppression of infections caused by *P. vivax, P. malariae,* and *P. ovale*?

    A. pyrimethamine-sulfadoxine
    B. hydroxychloroquine
    C. pyrimethamine
    D. primaquine
    E. chloroquine phosphate

19. Chloroquine phosphate is the drug of choice for the suppression of infections caused by strains of *P. falciparum* that are sensitive to chloroquine. The recommended adult dose is 300 mg base (500 mg salt) taken orally once a week beginning one to two weeks before entering a malarious area and continuing for

    A. one week after leaving the area
    B. three weeks after leaving the area
    C. six weeks after leaving the area
    D. nine weeks after leaving the area
    E. 12 weeks after leaving the area

20. Which of the following is the drug of choice to prevent delayed attacks of *P. vivax* and *P. ovale*?

    A. chloroquine phosphate
    B. pyrimethamine sulfadoxine
    C. hydrochloroquine
    D. pyrimethamine
    E. primaquine

21. Which of the following is the drug of choice to prevent clinical attacks in areas with chloroquine-resistant *P. falciparum*?

    A. pyrimethamine-sulfadoxine
    B. hydroxychloroquine
    C. primaquine
    D. pyrimethamine
    E. none of the above

22. Which of the following drugs has been tested thoroughly for safety and efficacy as prophylaxis against both chloroquine- and pyrimethamine-sulfadoxine-resistant strains of *P. falciparum*?

    A. quinine
    B. tetracycline
    C. hydroxychloroquine
    D. primaquine
    E. none of the above

23. Which of the following has not been found to have any harmful effect on the fetus when used in the recommended doses for malaria prophylaxis?

    A. chloroquine
    B. pyrimethamine
    C. tetracycline
    D. sulfa drugs
    E. quinine

24. Which of the following is the most common cause of death associated with measles?

    A. otitis media
    B. encephalitis
    C. pneumonia
    D. myocarditis
    E. thrombocytopenic purpura

25. There is evidence that smallpox vaccine has therapeutic value in the treatment of

    A. recurrent herpes simplex infection
    B. warts
    C. herpes zoster
    D. varicella
    E. none of the above

26. At the present time mortality is a reliable index of disease frequency in which of the following?

    A. coronary heart disease
    B. measles
    C. typhoid fever
    D. rabies
    E. poliomyelitis

27. Which of the following has not been implicated as a significant reservoir of rabies?

A. vampire bats
B. cats
C. rats (rodents)
D. foxes
E. guinea pigs

28. All of the following conditions transmitted by milk or milk products may be eliminated by pasteurization, *except*

    A. staphylococcal food poisoning
    B. brucellosis
    C. typhoid fever
    D. streptococcus A infections
    E. Q fever

29. Control of trichinosis for the foreseeable future will depend on

    A. detecting every infection in pigs by biopsy
    B. killing all larvae by radiation
    C. a safe, inexpensive drug that has no carryover into the meat
    D. detecting every infection in pigs by serologic methods
    E. thorough cooking of swine and other omnivorous or carnivorous animals

30. Which of the following is the most common form of chlorine to be used for water supply and waste water disinfection?

    A. chlorinated lime
    B. liquid chlorine
    C. calcium hypochlorite
    D. sodium hypochlorite
    E. chlorine dioxide

31. Patients with which of the following conditions should not be given live, attenuated virus vaccines?

    A. leukemia
    B. lymphoma
    C. congenital immune deficiency
    D. generalized malignancy
    E. all of the above

32. Immunity following vaccination seems to produce protection that lasts for at least four years in all of the following *except*

    A. cholera
    B. tetanus
    C. yellow fever
    D. poliomyelitis
    E. diphtheria

33. In which of the following diseases is there no evidence of temporary passive immunity in infants born of immune mothers?

    A. yellow fever
    B. rubella
    C. measles
    D. whooping cough
    E. diphtheria

34. In the United States there is no licensed vaccine against

    A. tetanus
    B. dengue
    C. yellow fever
    D. diphtheria
    E. cholera

35. Which of the following vaccinations is required to return to the United States?

    A. smallpox
    B. cholera
    C. yellow fever
    D. typhoid fever
    E. none of the above

36. At the present time the risk of vaccination is greater than the likelihood of the infection in

    A. pertussis
    B. diphtheria
    C. measles
    D. smallpox
    E. yellow fever

37. Which of the following is the most common life-threatening illness caused by *Hemophilus influenzae*?

    A. pneumonia
    B. meningitis
    C. acute otitis media
    D. septic arthritis
    E. sinusitis

38. A small area of redness will develop within 72 to 120 hours of injection of dilute diphtheria toxin. Reaction reaches its height after the fifth day, then gradually fades. This description corresponds with

   A. a positive Schick test
   B. a negative Schick test
   C. a positive Dick test
   D. a negative Dick test
   E. none of the above

39. A small area of redness will develop within 12 hours of injection of a small amount of suitable dilution of culture filtrate of a group A streptococcus. This description corresponds with

   A. a negative Dick test
   B. a positive Dick test
   C. a negative Schick test
   D. a positive Schick test
   E. none of the above

40. Which of the following is contraindicated in the treatment of ascariasis?

   A. piperazine compounds (Antepar)
   B. levamisole (Ketrax)
   C. pyrantel (Combatrin)
   D. thiabendazole
   E. tetrachloroethylene

41. Antitoxin is now used principally in the treatment of

   A. typhoid fever
   B. toxic shock syndrome
   C. diphtheria
   D. staphylococcal food poisoning
   E. mushroom poisoning

Directions: Each group of questions below consists of five lettered headings followed by a list of numbered words or phrases. For each numbered word or phrase select the one heading that is most closely related to it.

Questions 42 through 46

The usual avenue of emergence of the etiologic agent from the human host

   A. Saliva
   B. Feces or urine
   C. Skin lesions
   D. Bloodstream (by way of a biting arthropod)
   E. None of the above

42. typhoid fever
43. malaria
44. yaws (frambesia tropica, pian)
45. mumps
46. trachoma

Questions 47 through 51

   A. Susceptible
   B. Host
   C. Contact
   D. Reservoir of infectious agents
   E. Suspect

47. a person whose medical history and symptoms suggest that he or she may have or may be developing some communicable disease

48. a person or animal presumably not possessing sufficient resistance against a particular pathogenic agent to prevent contracting infection or disease if or when exposed to the agent

49. a person or animal that has been in an association with an infected person or animal or a contaminated environment that might provide an opportunity to acquire the infective agent

50. a person or other living animal, including birds and arthropods, that affords subsistence or lodgment to an infectious agent under natural (as opposed to experimental) conditions

51. any person, animal, arthropod, plant, soil, or substance (or combination of these) in which an infectious agent normally lives and multiplies, on which it depends primarily for survival, and in which it reproduces itself.

Questions 52 through 56

A. Enzootic
B. Epidemic
C. Epizootic
D. Endemic
E. Pandemic

52. present in a community at all times, but occurring in low frequency

53. more than the expected number of cases of a disease that would occur in a community or region during a given time period

54. present in a geographically defined animal community at all times at a relatively constant rate

55. the occurrence of a disease in a defined animal population, at a higher than expected rate

56. more than the expected number of cases of disease in widely scattered communities throughout the world

Questions 57 through 66

Incubation period

A. Less than 24 hours
B. One to seven days
C. About one to two weeks
D. Over two weeks
E. Unknown

57. thrush of infants *(Candida albicans)*
58. influenza
59. diphtheria
60. anthrax
61. herpangina
62. measles
63. pertussis
64. rubella
65. mumps
66. varicella

Questions 67 through 71

A. Rabies
B. Infectious hepatitis (viral hepatitis A)
C. Yellow fever
D. Serum hepatitis (viral hepatitis B)
E. Leprosy

Incubation period

67. usually two to eight weeks, occasionally as short as 10 days or as long as a year or more

68. three to six days

69. usually 45 to 160 days; average 60-90 days

70. from 15 to 50 days; average 28-30 days

71. the average is probably three to six years

Questions 72 through 76

A. *Aedes aegypti*
B. Anopheles
C. *Culex tarsalis*
D. Bugs
E. None of the above

72. dengue hemorrhagic fever
73. malaria
74. western equine encephalitis
75. Chagas' disease
76. yellow fever

Questions 77 through 81

A. Tsetse flies
B. Sandflies
C. Blackflies
D. Houseflies
E. Ticks

77. Rocky Mountain spotted fever
78. shigellosis
79. onchocerciasis (river blindness)
80. leishmaniasis
81. African trypanosomiasis

Questions 82 through 86

A. Incidence peaking from about two to six weeks of age
B. Incidence peaking from about three to four years of age
C. Incidence peaking from about 20 to 40 years of age
D. Incidence peaking from about 50 to 60 years of age
E. Bimodality of the age curve

82. tuberculosis
83. multiple sclerosis
84. Hodgkin's disease
85. hypertrophic pyloric stenosis
86. leukemia

Questions 87 through 91

A. Chloroquine
B. Primaquine
C. Quinine
D. Pyrimethamine-sulfadoxine
E. Tetracyclines

87. megaloblastic anemia, allergy, and disorders of the blood, kidney, liver, and nervous system
88. glucose-6-phosphate dehydrogenase (G6PD) deficiency should be ruled out by appropriate laboratory tests before administering this drug
89. tinnitus, headache, nausea, abdominal pain, photosensitivity, visual disturbance
90. gastrointestinal disturbance, headache, dizziness, severe retinopathy
91. severe intravascular hemolysis (blackwater fever)

Questions 92 through 96

A. Exanthem subitum (roseola infantum)
B. Measles (rubeola)
C. Scarlet fever (scarlatina)
D. German measles (rubella)
E. Erythema infectiosum (fifth disease)

92. febrile prodrome; cough, conjunctivitis, and coryza are usually marked; characteristic maculopapular rash
93. the onset of rash coincides with the disappearance of fever
94. fever; prominent postauricular and suboccipital nodes can be palpated
95. fever; painful tonsillopharyngitis; marked flushing of the cheeks and forehead that contrasts sharply with the characteristic circumoral pallor
96. absent or mild prodrome, confluent erythema, and edema of the cheeks (slapped face); central clearance of papular lesions (trunk and extremities) results in a striking rosette formation

Questions 97 through 101

A. Cytomegalovirus infections
B. Herpes simplex
C. Falciparum malaria
D. Viral hepatitis B (serum hepatitis)
E. Influenza

97. ecology of the disease affected by a cultural phenomenon (drug addiction)
98. an inverse correlation exists between its intensity (parasitemia) and the presence of the sickle cell trait
99. unique among infectious agents in its capacity to produce pandemics within a short period of time
100. activation has been a sequel of immunosuppressive drugs
101. prototype of latent infection that can be reactivated in later years in spite of demonstrable and persisting immunity

Questions 102 through 106

A. Group A coxsackievirus

36 / Public Health and Preventive Medicine Review

    B. Group B coxsackievirus
    C. Lymphocytic choriomeningitis
    D. Mumps virus
    E. Poliovirus

102. aseptic meningitis, herpangina (vesicular pharyngitis)

103. aseptic meningitis; hand, foot, and mouth disease (vesicular stomatitis with exanthem)

104. aseptic meningitis; three closely related but antigenically distinct virus strains

105. aseptic meningitis, epidemic pleurodynia, acute or subacute myocarditis or pericarditis

106. aseptic meningitis; fever, swelling, and tenderness of one or more salivary glands

Questions 107 through 111

    A. Postvaccinial encephalitis
    B. Progressive vaccinia (vaccinia necrosum)
    C. Eczema vaccinatum
    D. Generalized vaccinia
    E. Aberrant implantation of vaccinia

107. occurs in patients with immunologic defects; fever and systemic signs may be absent

108. autoinoculation of mucous membranes or abraded skin; more worrisome when occurring in the eye

109. very rare with current vaccine strains; apparently no established predisposing factor

110. usually minor illness with little residual damage; vesicles or pustules appear on normal skin distant from vaccination site

111. occurs in contacts as well as vaccinees; generally more severe in contact cases; patients frequently in a very toxic condition

Questions 112 through 116

Usual sources of common infections (or intoxications) transmitted by food

    A. Freshwater fish
    B. Rabbit meat
    C. Oysters
    D. Milk and egg products (custards, pastries)
    E. Honey

112. staphylococcal enteritis

113. botulism (infants)

114. clonorchiasis

115. tularemia

116. hepatitis A

Questions 117 through 121

    A. Cholera
    B. Milk sickness (alkali poisoning)
    C. Favism
    D. Ergotism
    E. Ciguatera

117. the onset is insidious, occurring after the ingestion of several meals of diseased bread

118. characterized by an excruciating sensation followed by gangrene of the extremities and other parts of the body

119. caused by consumption of the broad bean, which causes hemolysis in people with glucose-6-phosphate dehydrogenase deficiency

120. gastroenteritis, weakness, paresthesia, respiratory failure

121. the toxin bears resemblance to an anticholinesterase

Questions 122 through 126

    A. Varicella
    B. Diphtheria
    C. Typhoid fever
    D. Influenza
    E. Mumps (endemic parotitis)

122. respiratory obstruction, myocarditis, respiratory failure secondary to paralysis of the muscles of respiration due to neuritis

123. although uncommon in children, pneumonitis may occur in as many as 16% of adults

124. epididymo-orchitis, meningoencephalitis, hearing loss (frequently unilateral), pancreatitis

125. deaths result from the primary disease or from bacterial pneumonia; the aged and infirm are more vulnerable

126. infection of the gallbladder is common; spondylitis

Questions 127 through 131

    A. Sodium antimony gluconate
    B. Chloramphenicol
    C. Praziquantel
    D. Streptomycin
    E. None of the above

127. visceral leishmaniasis (kala azar)

128. schistosomiasis (*S. haematobium*)

129. tularemia

130. diphtheria

131. typhoid fever

Questions 132 through 136

    A. Amphotericin B (Fungizone)
    B. Potassium iodide
    C. Arsenic (trivalent)
    D. Penicillin
    E. Arsenic (pentavalent)

132. disseminated or chronic pulmonary cases of histoplasmosis

133. invasive forms of aspergillosis

134. lymphocutaneous infection of sporotrichosis

135. actinomycosis

136. disseminated infections of coccidioidomycosis

Questions 137 through 141

    A. Anthrax
    B. Brucellosis
    C. Leptospirosis
    D. Psittacosis (ornithosis)
    E. Tularemia

137. occurs in persons in occupations where there is contact with rats: sewermen, miners, rice and sugar field workers

138. an occupational disease in the tanning, gelatin, and animal hair and wool processing industries

139. an occupational disease of abattoir workers, livestock producers, veterinarian and laboratory workers; sporadic cases among consumers of unpasteurized milk

140. an occupational hazard to workers in the pet bird industry and in turkey processing plants

141. an occupational hazard to laboratory workers, hunters, farmers, and meat-market employees who handle wild rabbits

Questions 142 through 146

    A. Tetanus
    B. Tuberculosis
    C. Smallpox
    D. Measles
    E. Paratyphoid

142. most persons born in the United States before 1975 are likely to have been infected naturally and generally need not be considered susceptible

143. a traveler who anticipates possible prolonged exposure should have a skin test before leaving and a repeat test after returning to the United States

144. vaccination of civilians is indicated only for laboratory workers directly involved with the etiologic agent or closely related agents

145. primary immunization with a booster every 10 years is a universal recommendation regardless of age

146. vaccine effectiveness has never been established; food-borne rather than water-borne illness

Public Health and Preventive Medicine Review

Questions 147 through 151

 A. Mouse–mite–man
 B. Rodents–tick–man
 C. Rat–flea–man
 D. Man–louse–man
 E. None of the above

147. epidemic typhus fever (typhus exanthematicus); classical typhus fever

148. rickettsialpox

149. endemic typhus fever

150. trench fever

151. sodoku

Questions 152 through 156

 A. Epidemic (louse-borne) typhus
 B. Rocky Mountain spotted fever
 C. Endemic (flea-borne) typhus
 D. Q (query) fever
 E. Rickettsialpox

152. negative Weil-Felix reaction; only rickettsial infection characterized by vesiculation

153. positive Weil-Felix reaction with proteus OX-19; the disease may recrudesce years after the primary attack (Brill-Zinsser disease)

154. negative Weil-Felix reaction; pneumonitis is the best-known feature

155. positive Weil-Felix reaction with proteus OX-19 and OX-2; rash occurs first on hands and feet, wrists, and ankles

156. positive Weil-Felix reaction with proteus OX-19; *Rickettsia typhi* (mooseri)

Questions 157 through 161

 A. Agent is passed through the ovum from one mite generation to the next
 B. Agent is passed through the ovum from one tick generation to the next
 C. Agent can multiply in the free state
 D. Inevitably kills the infected vector
 E. None of the above

157. scrub typhus

158. Rocky Mountain spotted fever

159. tularemia

160. staphylococci

161. epidemic typhus

Questions 162 through 166

 A. Anthrax
 B. Pneumococcal pneumonia
 C. Diphtheria
 D. Herpes simplex
 E. Rabies

162. highly resistant spores in unfavorable conditions

163. metachromatic granules in internal structure of organism

164. the capsular material is a polysaccharide essential to its pathogenicity

165. causative agent may remain latent in cells until some specific stimulus initiates multiplication

166. cytoplasmatic Negri bodies

Questions 167 through 171

 A. Taeniasis (*Taenia saginatum*)
 B. Cysticercocis (larval stage of *Taenia solium*)
 C. Hydatidosis (*Echinococcus granulosis, E. multilocularis*)
 D. Diphyllobothriasis (*Diphyllobothrium latum*)
 E. Hymenolepiasis (*Hymenolepis nana*)

167. pork tapeworm disease

168. dog tapeworm disease

169. beef tapeworm disease

170. dwarf tapeworm disease

171. fish tapeworm disease

Questions 172 through 176

A. Actinomycosis
B. Coccidiodomycosis
C. Cryptococcosis
D. Sporotrichosis
E. Chromoblastomycosis

172. an important disease among migrant workers, archeologists, and military personnel from nonendemic areas who move into endemic areas (arid and semiarid areas)

173. often an occupational disease of farmers, gardeners, and horticulturists; the lymphatic type with linear cutaneous granulomas is the most common

174. a mycosis usually presenting as a subacute or chronic meningoencephalitis; susceptibility is increased in disorders of the reticuloendothelial system, particularly Hodgkin's disease

175. a chronic disease most frequently localized in the jaw, thorax, or abdomen; an occupational disease among persons who handle cattle; "sulfur granules," "lumpy jaw"

176. a chronic spreading mycosis of the skin and subcutaneous tissues, usually of a lower extremity; cauliflowerlike tumor

Directions: Each set of lettered headings below is followed by a list of numbered words or phrases. For each numbered word or phrase select

A. if the item is associated with A only
B. if the item is associated with B only
C. if the item is associated with both A and B
D. if the item is associated with neither A nor B

Questions 177 through 181

A. *Plasmodium falciparum* malaria
B. *Plasmodium vivax* malaria
C. Both
D. Neither

177. man is the only important reservoir

178. may be transmitted by blood transfusion

179. congenital transmission occurs

180. the clinical feature of this infection the paroxysms of fever occur day

181. fatal form of malaria that can kill a nonimmune person within a week or two of a primary attack unless appropriate treatment is given in time

Questions 182 through 186

A. Measles (rubeola)
B. Rubella (German measles)
C. Both
D. Neither

182. a red enanthem with surrounding pallor; may appear on the buccal mucosa two days prior to onset of rash

183. subacute sclerosing panencephalitis

184. lymphadenopathy is common, particularly of the occipital, posterior cervical, and postauricular lymph nodes

185. subclinical infection is common

186. maculopapular rash

Questions 187 through 191

A. Chickenpox (varicella)
B. Smallpox (variola)
C. Both
D. Neither

187. lesions appear in crops over a period of several days to one week

188. centripetal distribution of lesions more numerous on the body than on the limbs

189. involves palms and soles

190. under favorable conditions the virus may survive in crusts for as long as one year

191. deep-seated pox with infiltrated base

Public Health and Preventive Medicine Review

Questions 192 through 196

    A. Viral hepatitis A (infectious hepatitis)
    B. Viral hepatitis B (serum hepatitis)
    C. Both
    D. Neither

192. fecal oral transmission has not been demonstrated

193. homologous immunity follows infection

194. asymptomatic infections are more common in childhood than in adult life

195. the primary reservoir is man

196. specific treatment: none

Questions 197 through 201

    A. Inactivated polio virus vaccine (IPV)
    B. Oral polio virus vaccine (OPV)
    C. Both
    D. Neither

197. vaccine of choice for primary immunization of children in the United States

198. should not be used for immunizing immuno-deficient patients and their household contacts

199. possibility of hypersensitivity reactions to streptomycin and neomycin

200. confers passive protection

201. vaccine-associated poliomyelitis

Questions 202 through 206

    A. Water-borne
    B. Milk-borne
    C. Both
    D. Neither

202. typhoid fever

203. viral hepatitis A (infectious hepatitis)

204. bacillary dysentery (shigellosis)

205. brucellosis (undulant fever)

206. diphtheria

Questions 207 through 211

    A. Water-borne
    B. Milk-borne
    C. Both
    D. Neither

207. bovine tuberculosis

208. staphylococcal enterotoxin

209. streptococcal sore throat

210. amebic dysentery

211. giardiasis

Questions 212 through 216

    A. Amebic dysentery
    B. Bacillary dysentery (shigellosis)
    C. Both
    D. Neither

212. pyrexia rare unless complicated

213. complications: hepatic and other abscesses

214. mucous membrane not inflamed

215. tenesmus very severe

216. acute onset

Questions 217 through 221

    A. Staphylococcal food poisoning
    B. Botulism (adults)
    C. Both
    D. Neither

217. the most common form of food poisoning in the United States

218. attacks chiefly the central nervous system with only minor gastrointestinal symptoms

219. thermolabile toxin

220. the most potent poison known to mankind

221. an intoxication (not an infection)

Questions 222 through 226

    A. Active immunization (antigenic preparations, or vaccines)
    B. Passive immunization (globulin preparations, or antisera)
    C. Both
    D. Neither

222. chickenpox
223. mumps
224. rubella
225. typhoid fever
226. yellow fever

Questions 227 through 231

    A. Active immunization (antigenic preparations, or vaccines)
    B. Passive immunization (globulin preparations, or antisera)
    C. Both
    D. Neither

227. influenza
228. diphtheria
229. tetanus
230. rabies
231. measles

Questions 232 through 236

    A. Active immunization (antigenic preparations, or vaccines)
    B. Passive immunization (globulin preparations, or antisera)
    C. Both
    D. Neither

232. anthrax
233. tuberculosis
234. cholera
235. whooping cough
236. bubonic plague

Questions 237 through 241

    A. Rheumatic fever
    B. Acute poststreptococcal nephritis
    C. Both
    D. Neither

237. may leave residual cardiac damage
238. recurrent attacks may be frequent
239. mandatory antistreptococcal prophylaxis
240. most cases occur after skin infections
241. large epidemics have been reported

Questions 242 through 246

    A. *Ascaris lumbricoides*
    B. *Trichuris trichiuria*
    C. Both
    D. Neither

242. soil-transmitted helminth
243. human beings are the reservoir
244. Loeffler's syndrome (irregular respiration, spasms of coughing, fever, and pronounced blood eosinophilia)
245. diagnosis is made by identifying eggs in feces
246. migration through the lung of its host is required

Directions: For each of the incomplete statements below, ONE or MORE of the completions given is correct. In each case select

    A. if only 1, 2, and 3 are correct
    B. if only 1 and 3 are correct
    C. if only 2 and 4 are correct
    D. if only 4 is correct
    E. if all are correct

247. The persistently infected human host may remain infected for life and be continuously infective

    1. herpes simplex
    2. poliomyelitis
    3. influenza
    4. typhoid fever

248. Which of the following diseases is (are) quarantinable?
   1. cholera
   2. plague
   3. yellow fever
   4. smallpox

249. The term carrier refers to which of the following?
   1. incubatory carriers (persons who are excreting the agent before onset of illness)
   2. convalescent carriers
   3. chronic carriers
   4. persons with inapparent infections

250. The reservoir is animals in
   1. taeniasis
   2. rabies
   3. salmonellosis
   4. viral encephalitis

251. Human beings are the only known reservoir for
   1. diphtheria
   2. typhoid fever
   3. measles
   4. meningococcal meningitis

252. Human beings are important alternate hosts for the survival of the etiologic agent of
   1. yellow fever
   2. herpes simplex
   3. paratyphoid bacilli
   4. syphilis

253. The house fly is known to become contaminated with
   1. type A hepatitis
   2. salmonellosis
   3. ascaris
   4. anthrax

254. Transplacental infection may occur in
   1. moniliasis
   2. toxoplasmosis
   3. trichomoniasis
   4. vaccinia

255. The human infection would almost certainly become a "dead end" for the etiologic agent of
   1. tularemia
   2. murine typhus
   3. rabies
   4. St. Louis encephalitis

256. There is but a single target (organ or system) in the human body for the causative agent of
   1. rabies
   2. syphilis
   3. poliomyelitis
   4. tuberculosis

257. Surveys of seroimmunity (serologic epidemiology) have contributed greatly to the understanding of the epidemiology of
   1. tuberculosis
   2. yellow fever
   3. gonorrhea
   4. poliomyelitis

258. Known instances of the transmission of disease by infected persons on international flights have occurred with
   1. measles
   2. typhoid fever
   3. influenza
   4. bacillary dysentery

259. Relapses can occur in which of the following?
   1. *Plasmodium vivax* infections
   2. *Plasmodium falciparum* infections
   3. *Plasmodium ovale* infections
   4. *Plasmodium malariae* infections

260. Which of the following can be cured by drugs that are active only against the parasites' erythrocytic stages?
   1. *Plasmodium ovale* infections
   2. *Plasmodium malariae* infections

3. *Plasmodium vivax* infections
4. *Plasmodium falciparum* infections

261. Most pathogenic viruses are sensitive to
    1. markedly acid environment
    2. heat
    3. markedly alkaline environment
    4. low temperature

262. Aseptic meningitis may be caused by
    1. mumps virus
    2. polioviruses
    3. enteroviruses
    4. measles virus

263. The epidemiology of influenza is characterized by
    1. epidemic–pandemic potentiality
    2. high morbidity and low mortality
    3. "excess mortality" among predictably high-risk groups
    4. periodic–cyclic recurrences

264. Fever is a commonly reported symptom in
    1. botulism
    2. *Clostridium perfringens* food poisoning
    3. staphylococcal toxin poisoning
    4. salmonellosis

265. Trichinosis is characterized by
    1. the sudden appearance of edema of the upper eyelids
    2. remittent fever
    3. respiratory and neurologic symptoms
    4. marked eosinophilia

266. Which of the following is (are) involved in the maintenance of human trichinella infections in the United States?
    1. rats
    2. dogs
    3. cats
    4. swine

267. Chemoprophylaxis is used for the prevention of
    1. malaria
    2. meningococcal outbreak
    3. streptococcal outbreaks
    4. pinta

268. Recent administration of immune globulin or hyperimmune globulin can interfere with the response to
    1. mumps vaccine
    2. measles vaccine
    3. rubella
    4. rabies vaccine

269. Individuals with anaphylactic hypersensitivity to eggs should not be given
    1. live attenuated measles vaccine
    2. live attenuated mumps vaccine
    3. live attenuated rubella vaccine
    4. influenza vaccine

270. There is no convincing evidence of risk to the fetus from vaccination of pregnant women against which of the following?
    1. measles
    2. rubella
    3. mumps
    4. diphtheria

271. There is no special contraindication for vaccinating breast-feeding mothers with
    1. yellow fever vaccine
    2. diphtheria toxoid
    3. rubella vaccine
    4. tetanus toxoid

272. Vaccination against which of the following is (are) not required by any country as a condition for entry?
    1. typhus fever (epidemic louse-borne)
    2. plague
    3. meningococcal disease
    4. yellow fever

273. Vaccination is protective only against small infecting inocula; periodic single reinforcing injections are desirable, commonly once in three years for

1. diphtheria
2. yellow fever
3. poliomyelitis
4. typhoid fever

274. In which of the following disease(s) is active immunization produced by toxoids?

1. diphtheria
2. measles
3. tetanus
4. rubella

275. Infection does not confer effective immunity against

1. chickenpox
2. tetanus
3. smallpox
4. trachoma

276. The persistence of immunity following infection is lifelong and does not depend on reinfection in order to be maintained in which of the following?

1. treated syphilis
2. measles
3. gonorrhea
4. yellow fever

277. Systemic manifestations of meningococcal meningitis include

1. arthritis
2. pericarditis
3. pneumonia
4. meningitis

278. Diphtheria is an acute infectious disease of the

1. tonsils
2. pharynx
3. larynx
4. skin

Answers and Explanations
Epidemiology

1. **D.** At the World Health Assembly in May of 1980, the World Health Organization (WHO) declared the global eradication of smallpox. There is no evidence of smallpox transmission anywhere in the world. The last reported case of endemic smallpox occurred in Somalia in October 1977, and the last reported case of laboratory-acquired smallpox occurred in the United Kingdom in 1978. The World Health Organization amended the International Health Regulations on January 1, 1982 to delete smallpox from the diseases subject to regulation. (9:87)

2. **C.** Malaria is still the leading cause of death in the world. In India no fewer than 75 million persons suffer from it every year, and during epidemic years the incidence may reach twice that or even more. In Liberia, 90% of the children under five years of age have positive blood smears and 70% of the adults are continuously infected. Malaria is a constant scourge of a large part of the lowlands of South and Central America, large parts of Africa, and almost all of South and Southeast Asia. Leriche estimates a worldwide burden of 362,000 deaths and an annual incidence of about 25 million new cases; a prevalence of about 200 million is commonly considered. The latter represents about one out of every 20 people in the world. (20:35)

3. **B.** Generation time. (37:68)

4. **C.** The incubation period in human beings for rabies is usually two to eight weeks, occasionally as short as 10 days, or as long as a year or more; it depends on the severity of the wound, the site of the wound in relation to richness of nerve supply and distance from the brain, the amount of virus introduced, protection provided by clothing, and other factors. (6:274)

5. **D.** In measles, excretion of the agent terminates before clinical recovery; in diphtheria it may continue for some time after full recovery; in typhoid fever about 3% of all cases, in the absence of intervention, remain life-long carriers. In mumps, the virus may be excreted from seven days before to nine days after the clinical onset of disease. (37:68)

6. **E.** The attack rate is between 1 and 5% of people exposed. The incubation period averages five to six days and the mortality rate is approximately 15%. (19:229)

7. **E.** Carriers play an important role in the epidemiology of poliomyelitis, meningococcal meningitis, typhoid fever, and diphtheria. (30:26)

8. **E.** Inapparent infection is the presence of infection in a host without recognizable clinical signs or symptoms. Inapparent infections are only identifiable by laboratory means or by the development of positive reactivity to specific skin tests. Synonyms: asymptomatic, subclinical, or occult infection. Few infectious agents (measles is one) fail to produce a significant proportion of inapparent infections. Mumps is a generalized infection, with up to one third of infections being inapparent. It has been estimated that ordinarily not more than one in 500 persons who harbor pneumococci in the course of a year develops pneumonia. Poliomyelitis has a wide range of severity, from inapparent infection to paralysis and death. (6:412)

9. **C.** There is no evidence of spread of poliomyelitis from animals to human beings. Clonorchiasis results from eating fresh water fish containing encysted larvae. Echinococcosis is transmitted by hand-to-mouth transfer of dog feces and objects soiled with dog feces. Man acquires diphyllobothriasis by eating raw or inadequately cooked fish. Ingestion of viable cysts attached to grass and water plants, predominantly fresh watercress, leads to infection. (6:266)

45

10. **E.** Many disease agents require no insect vector to reach man. These include bacteria such as the salmonellae; the viruses of cowpox, rabies, and psittacosis; and animal parasites such as canine hookworm (the cause of creeping eruption). (6:417)

11. **C.** Weil's disease results from contact of the skin, especially if abraded, with water, moist soil, or vegetation contaminated with urine of infected animals. (6:194)

12. **E.** Hepatitis is the most important disease transmitted by blood transfusions. Cytomegalovirus disease, syphilis, and toxoplasmosis have also been transmitted by blood transfusion. (6:101)

13. **A.** *Escherichia coli* (20.2%). (37:295)

14. **A.** The urinary tract (40.6%). (37:292)

15. **E.** In brucellosis the white count is usually normal to low. Leucopenia is usual in measles, typhoid fever, and yellow fever. (6:31)

16. **E.** The risk of acquiring malaria is not uniform from country to country, or even within a country, and depends on local conditions. (10:4s)

17. **E.** The release of merozoites from erythrocytes initiates the chills and fever of a typical malaria paroxysm. (10:3s)

18. **E.** Chloroquine phosphate is the drug of choice for the suppression of infections caused by *P. vivax, P. malariae, P. ovale,* and the strains of *P. falciparum* that are sensitive to chloroquine. (10:18s)

19. **C.** Chloroquine phosphate is given in a dose of 300 mg base (500 mg salt) once a week, one to two weeks before, during, and for six weeks after a stay in malarious areas. (10:20s)

20. **E.** Primaquine is the drug of choice to prevent delayed attacks of *P. vivax* and *P. ovale.* It is not recommended for all travelers returning from malarious areas, and it should be given only after returning home. (10:19s)

21. **A.** Pyrimethamine-sulfadoxine is the drug of choice to prevent clinical attacks in areas with chloroquine-resistant *Plasmodium falciparum.* The drug is sold under the trade names Fansidar and Falcidar. Fansidar was licensed for sale in the United States in 1982. In addition to pyrimethamine-sulfadoxine, travelers should continue to take chloroquine weekly as the prophylactic drug of choice for non-*falciparum* species of malaria. (10:23s)

22. **E.** There is no drug currently available that has been tested thoroughly for safety and efficacy against these strains of *P. falciparum*. (10:25s)

23. **A.** Pregnancy is not a contraindication to malaria prophylaxis with chloroquine or another 4-aminoquinoline. Pyrimethamine is teratogenic in laboratory animals and its safety in human pregnancy is uncertain. Both tetracycline and quinine are contraindicated in pregnancy. The use of sulfa drugs late in pregnancy may be associated with neonatal jaundice. (10:26s)

24. **C.** Pneumonia is usually a result of secondary bacterial infection and is the most common cause of death associated with measles. Otitis media is another common complication, and encephalitis is a serious complication. Less common complications include thrombocytopenic purpura, mesenteric adenitis, kerato conjunctivitis, sinusitis, mastoiditis, and myocarditis. (37:135)

25. **E.** Smallpox vaccine should never be used therapeutically. There is no evidence that vaccination has therapeutic value in the treatment of any disease. (9:87)

26. **D.** Several requirements must be satisfied for mortality to be used as an index of time trends in disease occurrence. Most important, the disease must result in fatal outcome with uniform and significant frequency. When death occurs in less than 5% of cases or—as with measles—only once in 1,000 or more cases, mortality is an insensitive index of disease frequency. It is an unreliable index when improved treatment reduces case fatality, as with typhoid fever after chloramphenicol became available or with coronary heart disease since the introduction of intensive cardiac care units in many hospitals. Mortality is most reliable when case fatality rate is very high, as with human rabies. In the past, once clinical rabies developed, there was no known treatment to prevent death, but with massive medical support, two survivals have been documented. (12:272)

27. **C.** Rabies is not endemic in rodents. Bites by rats, mice, squirrels, rabbits, and other rodents have never been proved to produce human rabies, although, theoretically, that possibility exists. Rabies is transmitted to man through the bite of clinically rabid animals, primarily wild animals: skunk, fox, raccoon. In the lesser developed countries, dogs remain the principal reservoir. In some regions, transmission from infected vampire bats to domestic animals is common. (12:272)

28. **A.** The heat-stable enterotoxin of the staphylococci is not eliminated from milk by pasteurization if already present, although the staphylococci are destroyed. (27:223)

29. **E.** The private slaughter of pigs and home preparation of meat products that require little or no cooking are commonly responsible for outbreaks involving single families or small groups. (42:194)

30. **B.** Liquid chlorine is still by far the most common form of chlorine to be used for water supply and waste water disinfection. (37:999)

31. **E.** Similarly, patients receiving corticosteroids, alkylating agents, anti-metabolites, or radiation should not be given such vaccines. (9:63)

32. **A.** In cholera the duration of immunity is obscure, as indeed is the degree of protection afforded by this vaccine. In tetanus, the toxoid gives prolonged immunity, demonstrated for at least 10 years after a primary course of two doses and one reinforcing dose, using a potent toxoid. In yellow fever, the immunity lasts for 12 years and probably for life. Live poliovirus vaccine, using strains developed early in the history of these vaccines, has been shown to produce antibodies that were still present after 10 years. Diphtheria toxoid might well be expected to do the same as tetanus toxoid, although evidence based on the serum antitoxin level is limited to about four years. (6:80)

33. **D.** In whooping cough, maternal antibody crosses the placenta but does not protect infants against the disease. (23:237)

34. **B.** There is no licensed vaccine against dengue. (9:71)

35. **E.** No vaccinations are required to return to the United States. (9:8)

36. **D.** At the present time the small risk of vaccination is greater than the likelihood of infection with smallpox. (25:349)

37. **B.** Meningitis is the most common life-threatening illness caused by *Haemophilus influenzae*. (37:198)

38. **A.** A positive Schick test results from the irritative effect of toxin on the skin in the absence of a protective level of antitoxin in the bloodstream. This test has largely been replaced by direct measurement of serum antitoxin levels by the hemagglutination test. (37:186)

39. **B.** Before an attack of scarlet fever the intradermal injection of toxin results in an area of erythema appearing 8 to 24 hours later; after scarlet fever, because of antitoxin, no erythema appears at the test site. (37:176)

40. **E.** Tetrachloroethylene has been used in the past but, because of the suspicion that it might cause intestinal obstruction by agitating the worms into an entangled bolus, its use for ascariasis has been largely discontinued. (35:184)

41. **C.** If diphtheria is suspected, antitoxin should be given without awaiting bacteriologic confirmation. (6:117)

42. **B.** Culture of feces may be positive in half of the cases in the first week of fever and is more frequently positive in the second and third weeks of untreated disease. Bacteria may be passed in the urine, especially in the first weeks of illness. (37:226)

43. **D.** The agent may escape from the bloodstream by way of a biting female anophele mosquito. (37:68)

44. **C.** Most important in the transmission of yaws is the close bodily contact of a susceptible person, usually a child, with a patient with infectious lesions. (37:239)

45. **A.** The usual source of infection in mumps is the saliva. (37:146)

46. **E.** Transmission is through direct contact with ocular discharges and possibly mucoid or purulent discharges of nasal mucous membranes of infected persons, or through materials soiled therewith. Flies may contribute to the spread of the disease. (6:359)

47. **E.** This is the definition of suspect. (6:417)

48. **A.** This is the definition of susceptible. (6:417)

49. **C.** This is the definition of contact. (6:410)

50. **B.** This is the definition of host. (6:411)

51. **D.** This is the definition of reservoir. (6:416)

52. **D.** This is the definition of endemic. (10:100)

53. **B.** This is the definition of epidemic. (10:100)

54. **A.** This is the definition of enzootic. (10:100)

55. **C.** This is the definition of epizootic. (10:100)

56. **E.** This is the definition of pandemic. (17:242)

57. **B.** In moniliasis the incubation period is variable: two to five days in thrush of infants. (6:66)

58. **B.** Influenza: The incubation period is usually 24 to 72 hours. (6:177)

59. **B.** Diphtheria: The incubation period is usually two to five days, but occasionally is longer. (6:115)

60. **B.** Anthrax manifests within seven days—usually two to five. (6:13)

61. **B.** Herpangina: The incubation period is usually three to five days for herpangina and hand, foot, and mouth disease. (6:97)

62. **C.** Measles: The incubation period is about 10 days, varying from eight to 13 days from the time of exposure to onset of fever. (6:212)

63. **C.** Pertussis manifests almost uniformly within 10 days of exposure and not exceeding 21 days. (6:396)

64. **D.** Rubella manifests from 16 to 18 days after exposure, with a range of 14 to 21 days. (6:297)

65. **D.** Mumps: The incubation period is about two to three weeks and commonly 18 days. (6:232)

66. **D.** Varicella: The incubation period is from two to three weeks and commonly 13 to 17 days; this may be prolonged after passive immunization against varicella or in the immunodeficient. (6:76)

67. **A.** The incubation period for rabies is from two to eight weeks; it may be longer in vaccinated individuals. (6:74)

68. **C.** Yellow fever manifests within three to six days from exposure. (6:32)

69. **D.** Serum hepatitis: The incubation period is usually 45 to 160 days, the average 60–90 days, and it may be as short as two weeks and rarely as long as six to nine months; the variation is related in part to the amount of virus in the inoculum and the mode of transmission, as well as to host factors. (6:166)

70. **B.** Infectious hepatitis: The incubation period is from 15 to 50 days, depending on dose; the average is 28–30 days. (6:162)

71. **E.** Leprosy: The shortest known incubation period is seven months. The average is probably three to six years, although many years may elapse before the disease is recognized. (6:191)

72. **A.** Dengue hemorrhagic fever is transmitted by the bite of an infected *Aedes aegypti* mosquito. (36:270)

73. **B.** Malaria is transmitted by an infective female anopheline mosquito. (36:206)

74. **C.** In western equine encephalitis the arbovirus is carried by *Culex tarsalis*. (36:265)

75. **D.** The vectors of trypanosoma cruzi are large, nocturnal, blood-sucking reduviids. Both sexes and all stages are infected. (37:384)

76. **A.** Yellow fever is transmitted in urban and certain rural areas by the bite of infective *Aedes aegypti* mosquitoes. (37:342)

77. **E.** Rocky Mountain spotted fever is ordinarily transmitted by the bite of an infected tick. (6:292)

78. **D.** There is abundant circumstantial evidence that houseflies *(M. domestica)*, where they are numerous, are important carriers of shigellae from the feces of infected persons to other people, perhaps largely by contaminating food. (36:373)

79. **C.** Onchocerca volvulus is transmitted by blackflies of the *Similium* genus. (36:166)

80. **B.** Leishmaniasis is caused by parasites of the genus *Leishmania*. They are transmitted by sandflies. (36:93)

81. **A.** There is no evidence that biting flies other than the tsetse are concerned in the spread of human trypanosomiasis. (36:73)

82. **E.** The occurrence of two or more peaks in an age curve suggests that different etiologic factors may be involved in the disease as it occurs at different ages, even if the clinical and pathologic manifestations of the disease are the same at all ages. (12:61)

83. **C.** The age trend of multiple sclerosis, with incidence peaking between 20 and 40 years of age, is so unlike that of any other chronic disease that it demands explanation. (12:61)

84. **E.** (12:61)

85. **A.** Hypertrophic pyloric stenosis of infancy has perhaps the most restricted age range of any postnatal disease. (12:61)

86. **E.** Bimodality of age curve is seen in tuberculosis, leukemia, and Hodgkin's disease. (12:61)

87. **D.** The use of pyrimethamine in high doses or for prolonged periods may cause hematologic toxicity, including megaloblastic anemia due to folate deficiency. (10:24s)

88. **B.** Before any use of primaquine, G6PD deficiency should be ruled out by appropriate laboratory tests. It can result in hemolysis. (10:22s)

89. **C.** Reactions to quinine frequently occur in the form of cinchonism. (10:25s)

90. **A.** When chloroquine is used in high doses for prolonged periods, as in the treatment of rheumatoid arthritis, it may cause a severe retinopathy characterized by loss of central visual acuity, pigmentation of the macula, and constriction of the retinal artery. (10:19s)

91. **C.** The intermittent use of quinine has been associated with severe intravascular hemolysis (blackwater fever). (10:25s)

92. **B.** In measles, following the incubation period, the patient typically develops fever and malaise; coryza, conjunctivitis, and cough appear shortly thereafter. The characteristic maculopapular rash appears two to six days after the onset of fever and malaise. (37:135)

93. **A.** In exanthem subitum, a maculopapular rash on the trunk and later on the rest of the body ordinarily follows lysis of the fever. (6:299)

94. **D.** In rubella, postauricular, suboccipital, or postcervical lymphadenopathy are common but not pathognomonic; occasionally adenopathy is generalized. (6:295)

95. **C.** Scarlet fever is characterized by enanthem, strawberry tongue, exanthem. Typically the rash does not involve the face, but there is flushing of the cheeks and circumoral pallor. (6:332)

96. **E.** Erythema infectiosum manifests with striking erythema of the cheeks (slapped-face appearance) and reddening of the skin that fades and recurs; the body may show a lacelike serpeginous rash. (6:299)

97. **D.** Viral hepatitis is transmitted by contaminated needles, syringes, and other intravenous equipment—important vehicles of spread, especially among drug addicts. (6:166)

98. **C.** In falciparum malaria, persons with sickle cell trait have relatively lower parasitemia when infected with *P. falciparum*. (6:207)

99. **E.** Influenza pandemics during the last 90 years began in 1889, 1918, 1957, and 1968. (6:176)

100. **A.** With respect to cytomegalovirus infections, fetuses, patients with debilitating disease, or those on immunosuppressive drugs are more susceptible to overt and severe disease—especially renal transplant recipients. (6:101)

101. **B.** Herpes simplex virus is one of the most widely disseminated agents causing infections in man. Although antibodies to the virus develop, the virus is not eliminated from the body, and a carrier state (latent infection) is established that lasts throughout life and is associated with recurrent attacks of the disease. (37:168)

102. **A.** Coxsackievirus group A types: 2, 3, 4, 5, 6, 8, 10, and 22 for herpangina. (6:96)

103. **A.** Coxsackievirus group A types: 4, 5, 9, 10, and 16 (predominantly) for hand, foot, and mouth disease. (6:96)

104. **E.** Poliovirus types 1, 2, and 3 are classified as picornaviruses belonging to the enterovirus group. (37:146)

105. **B.** Group B coxsackievirus types 1–5 and echovirus 11 have been associated with these illnesses. (6:255)

106. **D.** Mumps virus is antigenically related to the parainfluenza viruses. (6:232)

107. **B.** Progressive vaccinia (vaccinia necrosum) occurs in individuals with immunologic defects or in those who are receiving immunosuppressive drugs, corticosteroids, or radiation therapy. (6:318)

108. **E.** When aberrant implantation of vaccinia occurs in the eyes, it is advisable to request treatment by an ophthalmologist. (6:318)

109. **A.** Postvaccinial encephalitis is believed to represent a hypersensitivity phenomenon rather than a central nervous system infection per se. (6:318)

110. **D.** This describes generalized vaccinia with multiple lesions on various parts of the body. (6:318)

111. **C.** Eczema vaccinatum occurs in those with past or present eczema, which may arise in eczematous siblings of vaccinees. (6:318)

112. **D.** Among the foods most susceptible to staphylococcal contamination are pastries, custards, salads. (57:35)

113. **E.** Honey, one food item fed to infants, often contains *Clostridium botulinum* spores. (6:62)

114. **A.** Clonorchiasis is a trematode disease of the bile ducts. Man becomes infected by eating raw

or partly cooked freshwater fish that harbor *Clonorchis sinensis*. (57:159)

115. **B.** Tularemia may be transmitted to humans by ingestion of insufficiently cooked meat of infected rabbit. (57:93)

116. **C.** Common-vehicle outbreaks have been related to contaminated water and food, including milk, sliced meats, salads, and raw or undercooked clams and oysters. (6:162)

117. **D.** Ergotism is caused by ergot *(Claviceps prupurea)*, a highly toxic fungus that grows on rye and other grains used in the making of bread. (57:167)

118. **D.** In ergotism, preceding the onset of gangrene, patients complain of weakness, headache, and convulsive depression. (57:167)

119. **C.** Favism results from consumption of or exposure to the pollen of broad bean, *Vicia fava*, which causes hemolysis in people with glucose-6-phosphate dehydrogenase deficiency. Males with this deficiency tend to suffer acute hemolytic reactions to drugs such as primaquine and to contact with broad beans. (57:213)

120. **E.** The syndrome of ciguatera usually consists of gastroenteritis for one or two days, weakness for two days to a week, and paresthesia for two days to three weeks. (35:545)

121. **E.** Ciguatoxin bears resemblance to an anticholinesterase. (35:545)

122. **B.** Toxin-related complications can follow inoculation of diphtheria at any anatomic site. (37:187)

123. **A.** It has been estimated that 16% to 33% of adults with chickenpox have clinical or radiologic evidence of pneumonitis. (37:147)

124. **E.** Epididymo-orchitis is a well-known complication of mumps infection. Hearing loss, which is frequently unilateral and often permanent, is estimated to occur once in every 15,000 patients with mumps. (37:145)

125. **D.** For centuries, the aged and infirm have been observed to be vulnerable to severe or fatal influenza. (37:116)

126. **C.** In typhoid fever, bacteria may be passed in the urine, especially during the first weeks of illness. Organisms are found in greater numbers in the gallbladder than in the feces and are also likely to be present in duodenal aspirates. (37:226)

127. **A.** Sodium antimony gluconate is effective in the treatment of visceral leishmaniasis. (6:189)

128. **C.** Praziquantel is the drug of choice against all three species of schistosoma. (6:307)

129. **D.** Streptomycin is the drug of choice in the treatment of tularemia. (6:381)

130. **E.** If diphtheria is suspected, antitoxin should be given without awaiting bacteriologic confirmation. Penicillin and erythromycin are effective against the organism but should be administered only after cultures are taken, in conjunction with but not as a substitute for antitoxin. (6:117)

131. **B.** Chloramphenicol is the drug of choice for acute typhoid fever. For strains not sensitive to it, other drugs such as ampicillin are of proven value. (6:385)

132. **A.** Amphotericin B is the drug of choice in the treatment of histoplasmosis. (36:497)

133. **A.** Amphotericin B should be tried in tissue-invasive forms of aspergillosis. Any immunosuppressive therapy in use should be reduced or discontinued. (6:54)

134. **B.** Potassium iodide is specific in lymphocutaneous infection of sporotrichosis. In other forms, amphotericin B is effective. (6:323)

135. **D.** Prolonged administration of penicillin in high doses is usually effective in the treatment of actinomycosis. Tetracyclines are second in choice. (6:2)

136. **A.** Treatment is indicated in the disseminated disease. Amphotericin B is active against *C. immitis* when given by intravenous route. Early experience with ketoconazole has been encouraging. (30:483)

137. **C.** Persons in occupations that involve exposure to water and mud carry a high risk for leptospiral infections. (37:423)

138. **A.** Anthrax is primarily an occupational hazard of workers who process hides, hair (especially from goats), bone and bone products, and wool. (6:12)

139. **B.** Brucellosis is primarily an occupational disease of those working with infected animals or their tissues, especially farm workers, veterinarians, and abattoir workers. (6:64)

140. **D.** Psittacosis outbreaks occasionally occur in individual households, pet shops, aviaries, and

pigeon lofts. Turkey and duck farms have been sources of disease. (6:240)

141. **E.** With respect to tularemia, certain occupations have traditionally been associated with high risk of infection. These include laboratory workers, trappers, hunters, farmers, sheep shearers, and meat market employees who handle wild rabbits. (37:48)

142. **D.** Persons can be considered immune to measles only if they have documentation of physician-diagnosed measles, laboratory evidence of measles immunity, or adequate immunization with live measles vaccine on or after the first birthday. (9:79)

143. **B.** Travelers who are already positive are unlikely to be reinfected (tuberculosis). (9:87)

144. **C.** Vaccination of civilians is indicated only for laboratory workers directly involved with smallpox or closely related (orthopox) viruses (e.g., monkeypox, vaccinia, and others). (9:87)

145. **A.** Since there is no natural immunity to the tetanus toxin and since the tetanus organism is found throughout the world, primary immunization with a booster every 10 years is a universal recommendation, regardless of age. (9:87)

146. **E.** The effectiveness of a paratyphoid vaccine has never been established. (9:89)

147. **D.** The body louse, *Pediculus humanus humanus*, is infected by feeding on the blood of a patient with acute typhus fever. Man is infected by rubbing feces or crushed lice into the bite or into superficial abrasions. (35:433)

148. **A.** Rickettsialpox is caused by *Rickettsia akari*, a member of the spotted fever group of rickettsiae transmitted to man from mice by a mite. (35:433)

149. **C.** In endemic typhus fever (murine typhus), infective rat fleas (usually *Xenopsylla cheopis*) defecate rickettsiae while sucking blood and contaminate the bite site and other fresh skin wounds. (35:433)

150. **D.** In trench fever, man is infected by inoculation of the organism in louse feces through a skin break from either the bite of the louse or other means. (35:433)

151. **E.** Sodoku (rat-bite) fever due to *Spirillum minor*) is usually caused by the bites of brown or black rats. (35:433)

152. **E.** The initial lesion of rickettsialpox resembles that of mite typhus, and the rash is similar to that of other members of this group, except that vesicles occur. (36:435)

153. **A.** Epidemic typhus may recrudesce years after the primary attack; this need not be associated with lice. (36:435)

154. **D.** Q fever may present as a variety of clinical syndromes: fever, endocarditis, and pericarditis. Pneumonitis is the best-known feature. (36:435)

155. **B.** In Rocky Mountain spotted fever, the rash appears from the fourth to the seventh day. It is seen as small rose-coloured spots resembling measles but soon becomes petechial, spreading to become confluent. (36:435)

156. **C.** Endemic (murine typhus) is usually milder than epidemic typhus. No Brill-Zinsser phenomenon has been observed. (36:435)

157. **A.** Transovarial passage of *R. orientalis* (the cause of scrub typhus) in the mite vector is essential to the cycle of transmission. (17:61)

158. **B.** The arthropod species itself constitutes a nearly complete reservoir mechanism when the agent is passed through the ovum from one arthropod generation to the next. This phenomenon has been observed in ticks infected with the rickettsial agent of Rocky Mountain spotted fever. (17:61)

159. **B.** This phenomenon has been observed in ticks infected with the bacillus of tularemia. (17:61)

160. **C.** Staphylococci can multiply in the free state. (17:62)

161. **D.** Infection of invertebrate species ordinarily endures for the life of the arthropod and has no influence on the life span, except for infection with *R. prowazekii* (epidemic typhus), which inevitably kills the infected vector (the human louse). (17:60)

162. **A.** Bacillus anthracis, the etiologic agent of anthrax, is a large, gram-positive, nonmotile, spore-forming bacterial rod. (37:425)

163. **C.** Metachromatic granules of *Corynebacterium diphtheria* are demonstrated when the bacilli are stained with a suitable preparation of methylene blue. (37:185)

164. **B.** The capsular material of *Streptococcus pneumoniae*, the pneumococcus, is a polysaccharide, the nature of which determines the type of organism and its pathogenicity. (37:201)

165. **D.** Although antibodies to the herpes simplex virus develop, the virus is not eliminated from the body, and a carrier state (latent infection) is established that lasts throughout life and is associated with recurrent attacks of the disease.
(37:168)

166. **E.** The virus can be identified by the development of Negri bodies in brain neurons. (37:410)

167. **B.** Infection with the adult or larval stage of the pork tapeworm, *Taenia solium*, is referred to as cysticercosis. (57:153)

168. **C.** In hydatidosis, the dog tapeworms *Echinococcus granulosus* and *Echinococcus multilocularis* are found not only in dogs but also in other members of the canidae family such as wolves and foxes. (57:155)

169. **A.** Taeniasis is an infection with the adult stage of the beef tapeworm, *Taenia saginatum*. (57:153)

170. **E.** A type of tapeworm that is more common in children than in adults is the dwarf tapeworm, known as *Hymenolepis nana*. (57:157)

171. **D.** Infection with the fish tapeworm, *Diphyllobothrium latum*, also known as the broad tapeworm, is a nonfatal disease of long duration, often with trivial or absent symptoms. (57:156)

172. **B.** The southwestern United States is an endemic area of coccidioidomycosis. Most patients acquiring the infection develop a positive skin test. (6:86)

173. **D.** An epidemic of sporotrichosis among gold miners in South Africa involved some 3,000 miners; the fungus was growing in mine timbers. (6:322)

174. **C.** The cause of death in cryptococcosis (torulosis) is generally central nervous system involvement. (6:99)

175. **A.** "Sulfur granules" are colonies of the infectious agent (actinomyces) (6:1)

176. **E.** Chromoblastomycosis is a chronic, spreading mycosis. Eventually large verrucous or even cauliflower masses and lymph stasis develop. (6:82)

177. **C.** Man is the only important reservoir of human malaria, although higher apes may harbor *P. malariae*. (6:206)

178. **C.** Malaria may also be transmitted by injection or transfusion of blood of infected persons or by use of contaminated hypodermic syringes, as by drug addicts. (6:206)

179. **C.** Congenital malaria occurs rarely. (6:206)

180. **D.** The clinical feature of *P. malariae* malaria (in the absence of multiple infections) is that the paroxysms of fever occur every fourth day. (35:53)

181. **A.** Various symptoms and clinical signs that often occur with *falciparum* infections are rarely, if ever, seen in other malarias (shock, renal failure, acute encephalitis, coma). (6:48)

182. **A.** These are called Koplick spots. (37:134)

183. **A.** Evidence indicates that measles virus is associated with a progressive degenerative disease of the brain: subacute sclerosing panencephalitis (Dawson encephalitis). (37:134)

184. **B.** Lymphadenopathy may appear three to five days before the rash and persist several days after the rash disappears (rubella). (37:140)

185. **B.** Subclinical infection is common in rubella and may occur in up to one third of infections. (37:140)

186. **C.** A maculopapular rash is seen in rubeola and rubella. (37:134)

187. **A.** Chickenpox spots appear in crops and in different stages of development. Smallpox spots appear together and are therefore at the same stage. (30:102)

188. **A.** Chickenpox rash tends to avoid limbs and is centripetal. Smallpox rash presents on limbs and is centrifugal. (30:102)

189. **B.** Smallpox involves the palms and soles. These areas are not often involved in chickenpox. (30:102)

190. **B.** The virus of smallpox can survive in crusts, under favorable conditions, for as long as a year, but chickenpox virus dies rapidly. (23:236)

191. **B.** Smallpox lesions are deep-seated, with an infiltrated base, circular, homogeneous, multilocular, and umbilicated. Secondary infection is usual. Chickenpox lesions are superficial and the base is not infiltrated; the lesions are often oval, not homogeneous, generally not loculated, and never umbilicated. Secondary infection is rare. (37:102)

192. **B.** Fecal-oral transmission has not been demonstrated (serum hepatitis). Person-to-person infection is by the fecal-oral route in infectious hepatitis. (6:166)

193. **C.** Homologous immunity after attack probably lasts for life. (6:162)

194. **C.** Infection with hepatitis B virus may occur with or without symptoms and, as with hepatitis A virus infection, asymptomatic infections are more common in childhood than in adult life. (37:160)

195. **C.** The primary reservoir of hepatitis B virus is man, although, as is the case with hepatitis A virus, evidence of naturally occurring infection has been found in chimpanzees. (37:162)

196. **C.** There is no specific treatment for infectious hepatitis or serum hepatitis. (6:164)

197. **B.** Trivalent oral polio vaccine (OPV) is the vaccine of choice for all infants, children, and adolescents (up to eighteenth birthday) in the United States, if there are not contraindications to vaccinations. (9:80)

198. **B.** Patients with immune deficiency diseases should not be given OPV because of their substantially increased risk of vaccine-associated disease. (9:81)

199. **A.** Since IPV contains traces of streptomycin and neomycin, there is a possibility of hypersensitivity reactions in individuals sensitive to these antibiotics. (9:81)

200. **D.** Both of them confer active protection. (9:80)

201. **D.** It has been estimated that one case of vaccine-associated disease occurs for every 3 to 4 million doses of OPV distributed. (37:152)

202. **C.** Typhoid fever may be transmitted by food or water contaminated by feces or urine of a patient or carrier. Vegetables, milk, and milk products are usually contaminated by the hands of carriers. (6:382)

203. **C.** Common-vehicle outbreaks of viral hepatitis A have been related to contaminated water and food, including milk, sliced meats, salads, and raw or undercooked clams and oysters. (6:162)

204. **C.** Water-, milk-, and fly-borne transmission of bacillary dysentery may occur as the result of direct fecal contamination. (6:308)

205. **B.** Brucellosis may be transmitted by ingestion of raw milk or dairy products. (6:64)

206. **B.** Raw milk has served as a vehicle of diphtheria. (6:115)

207. **B.** Bovine tuberculosis results from exposure to tuberculous cattle, usually by ingestion of unpasteurized milk or dairy products. (6:374)

208. **B.** Staphylococcal enterotoxin may be of bovine origin and transmitted by contaminated milk or milk products. (6:138)

209. **B.** Milk and milk products have been associated most frequently with food-borne outbreaks. (6:335)

210. **A.** Epidemics occur mainly as a result of contaminated water containing cysts from feces of infected persons. (6:3)

211. **A.** Localized outbreaks of giardiasis result from contaminated water supplies. (6:150)

212. **A.** Pyrexia is rare in amebic dysentery unless complicated. Pyrexia is common in bacillary dysentery. (36:375)

213. **A.** Complications of amebic dysentery include hepatic and other abscesses, amebiasis of skin, and perforation. Toxic arthritis and eye complications may result in bacillary dysentery. (36:375)

214. **A.** In amebic dysentery the mucous membranes are not inflamed; the bowel wall is thickened. In bacillary dysentery the membrane is hyperaemic and inflamed; the bowel wall is not thickened. (36:375)

215. **B.** Tenesmus is very severe in bacillary dysentery; tenesmus is not usual in amebic dysentery. (36:375)

216. **B.** The onset is acute in bacillary dysentery. There is an insidious onset in amebic dysentery. (36:375)

217. **A.** Staphylococcal food poisoning is the most common form of food poisoning in the United States. (57:34)

218. **B.** Botulism differs from other types of food-borne diseases in that it attacks chiefly the central nervous system, with only minor gastrointestinal symptoms. (57:50)

219. **B.** Unlike the toxin produced by staphylococci, botulinus toxin is thermolabile. Higher tempera-

tures, however, are required for the inactivation of the spores. (57:51)

220. **B.** The microorganism that causes botulism is a harmless saprophyte, but the toxin it produces is one of the most potent poisons known to mankind. The fatality rate for staphylococcal food poisoning is, for all practical purposes, negligible, while that for botulism is about 65% and higher when large quantities of the neurotoxin are ingested and absorbed. (57:50)

221. **C.** Staphylococcal food poisoning and botulism are intoxications. (57:34)

222. **B.** Chickenpox: Gamma globulin is effective in modifying or preventing disease if given 96 hours after exposure. (6:77)

223. **C.** Mumps: Live attenuated vaccine is available. Human immune globulin is of questionable effectiveness when administered following exposure but may be considered for pregnant women. (6:233)

224. **C.** Rubella: A single dose of attenuated rubella virus vaccine elicits a significant antibody response in approximately 95% of susceptibles. Immune serum globulin given after exposure early in pregnancy will not prevent infection or viremia in all cases but may modify or suppress symptoms. (6:297)

225. **A.** Typhoid fever: An inactivated suspension of *Salmonella typhi* is available as a vaccine. (36:636)

226. **A.** Yellow fever: A single subcutaneous injection of a vaccine containing viable ITD strain virus cultivated in chick embryo is effective. (36:636)

227. **A.** Influenza: Active immunization is effective when a sufficient mass of antigens closely matching the prevailing strain of virus is administered. (36:635)

228. **C.** Diphtheria: A toxoid is available for active immunization, and an antitoxin for passive immunization and treatment. (36:634)

229. **C.** Tetanus: A vaccine containing modified tetanus toxin (toxoid) and an antiserum containing an antitoxin are available. (36:636)

230. **C.** Rabies: A vaccine and an antiserum are available. (36:635)

231. **C.** Measles: Live attenuated vaccine is the agent of choice. For immediate prophylaxis human normal immunoglobulin may be given. (36:635)

232. **A.** Anthrax: Immunization of high-risk persons is recommended. The vaccine is effective in preventing cutaneous and probably inhalation anthrax. (6:13)

233. **A.** A suspension of living attenuated bacilli is available, which gives protection against tuberculosis. *Bacillus calmette-guerin* vaccine (BCG). (36:634)

234. **A.** A suspension of killed cholera vibrios of INABA and OGAWA strains is available, which gives a short-lived immunity. An el-tor vibrio vaccine is also available. (36:634)

235. **A.** A suspension of killed *Bordetella pertusis* for active immunity is available. (36:635)

236. **A.** A suspension of killed *Pasteurella pestis* is commonly used. Its value is uncertain. (36:635)

237. **A.** Since carditis is the only manifestation of rheumatic fever that can lead to permanent sequelae, interest in prevention of rheumatic fever focuses on this manifestation. Prognosis of acute glomerulonephritis: usually complete recovery. (37:184)

238. **A.** One of the most striking characteristics of rheumatic fever is its tendency to recur. Recurrent attacks are rare in acute glomerulonephritis. (37:184)

239. **A.** Because of the concern over recurrent attacks of rheumatic fever and in particular because of the likelihood of a recurrence aggravating the cardiac damage from preceding attacks, continuous antistreptococcal prophylaxis is essential. Persons who have had glomerulonephritis do not require continuous antistreptococcal prophylaxis. (37:184)

240. **B.** In many areas today, most cases of poststreptococcal glomerulonephritis occur after skin infections rather than throat infections. (37:184)

241. **B.** In contrast to rheumatic fever, acute poststreptococcal glomerulonephritis is seen in epidemic form. (37:184)

242. **C.** Ascaris is the chief of the so-called soil-transmitted helminths, a group that also includes trichuris, strongyloides, and hookworms. (37:473)

243. **C.** Human beings are the reservoir of *Ascaris lumbricoides* and *Trichuris trichiuria*. (6:366)

244. **A.** The passage of worms through the lungs, particularly in previously unexposed hosts, may pre-

cipitate a pneumonitis characterized by fever, cough, and high eosinophilia. (6:51)

245. **C.** Eggs are present in feces of infected persons. (6:366)

246. **A.** This describes the life cycle of *Ascaris lumbricoides*. (37:474)

247. **D.** The infected host may be continuously infective in typhoid fever. A relatively brief excretion period characterizes measles and influenza. Polioviruses are excreted on the average for about fifty days and may be excreted for three months or longer in individual instances. Herpes simplex is intermittently infective. (17:60)

248. **A.** Smallpox has been deleted from the quarantinable diseases. (9:VIII)

249. **E.** A carrier is a person who harbors the infective agents without showing signs of disease but is capable of transmitting the agent to other persons. (30:26)

250. **E.** The term zoonosis is applied to those infectious diseases of vertebrate animals that are transmissible to man under natural conditions. (37:27)

251. **E.** Man—patients and especially carriers—is the only reservoir of typhoid fever. Man is also the only reservoir of diphtheria, measles, and meningococcal meningitis. (6:382)

252. **B.** Human beings are important alternate hosts for the etiologic agent of yellow fever and paratyphoid bacilli. Human beings—the only host—are essential to the survival of the etiologic agent of herpes simplex and syphilis. (17:59)

253. **E.** The house fly is known to become contaminated with 100 species of pathogenic organisms. The nonbiting mouthparts are the key to this transmission. (37:505)

254. **C.** Transplacental infection of toxoplasmosis may occur in women with primary infection. Fetal vaccinia results from blood-borne dissemination of vaccinia virus in the pregnant woman given primary vaccination. Moniliasis may be transmitted from mother to infant during childbirth. Trichomoniasis may be transmitted by contact with vaginal and urethral discharges of infected persons. (6:356)

255. **E.** Human beings are incidental victims and play no role in the maintenance of the agent in nature. (17:59)

256. **B.** For some agents like polio or rabies viruses there is but a single vulnerable target, in these cases the central nervous system, whereas for other agents such as syphilis and tubercle bacillus, multiple targets exist. (17:187)

257. **C.** Sero surveys have contributed to the understanding of yellow fever and poliomyelitis. (17:286)

258. **E.** In the United States a traveler arriving from an infected area who has not met immunization requirements is given a "surveillance notice" specifying the disease to which he or she may have been exposed. (46:615)

259. **B.** Relapses occur when *P. vivax* or *P. ovale* parasites that have remained dormant in the liver for months or years mature, enter the blood, and initiate another series of erythrocytic cycles. (10:3s)

260. **C.** *P. malariae* and *P. falciparum* infections can be cured by drugs that are active only against the parasite's erythrocytic stages. In *P. ovale* and *P. vivax* infections, therapy directed at the erythrocytic stages may eliminate parasites from the blood but will not prevent relapses caused by parasites persisting in the liver. (10:3s)

261. **A.** Viruses are inactivated by high temperatures, similar to those used to kill bacteria. They withstand low temperatures and are preserved in deep freeze units at 70°C. A markedly acid or alkaline environment destroys most viruses. (8:187)

262. **E.** Aseptic meningitis is caused by a wide variety of infectious agents, many of which are associated with other specific diseases. (6:218)

263. **E.** Influenza is first an epidemic disease. There have been about 35 pandemics of influenza since 1510. Influenza is rarely fatal. Deaths attributed specifically to pneumonia and influenza (a reporting category) comprise only 25-50% of all excess deaths that occur during an epidemic. Epidemics caused by type A influenza viruses occur more frequently and cause greater excess mortality than type B epidemics. Generally, two to three years elapse between type A epidemics; three to six years elapse between type B epidemics. (37:115)

264. **D.** Fever is a commonly reported symptom in salmonellosis. Fever is typically absent in botulism, staphylococcal food poisoning, and *Clostridium perfringens* food poisoning. (37:307-14)

265. **E.** The clinical course of trichinosis in man is variable, depending on the numbers of larvae ingested and other factors. (6:236)

266. **E.** Rats, dogs, swine, and many wild animals. (6:363)

267. **E.** Mass administration of effective chemotherapeutic drugs to all members of a population without determining if they are infected has sometimes been dramatically effective. (37:81)

268. **A.** Recent administration of immune globulin (formerly called immune serum globulin (ISG) and immunoglobulin) or hyperimmune globulin can interfere with the response to live, attenuated virus vaccine. Therefore, administration of live, attenuated virus vaccines should be deferred until approximately three months after passive immunization. Inactivated vaccines are sometimes administered concurrently with passive antibody to induce active immunity, as is done for postexposure rabies prophylaxis. (9:64)

269. **D.** Influenza vaccine. This would include persons who, upon ingestion of eggs, develop swelling of the lips or tongue or who experience acute respiratory distress or collapse. Live, attenuated measles, mumps, or rubella vaccines prepared from viruses grown in cell cultures can be given safely regardless of a history of allergy to eggs or egg protein. (9:62)

270. **D.** On grounds of theoretical risk to the developing fetus, live, attenuated-virus vaccines are not generally given to pregnant women or to those likely to become pregnant with three months after vaccination. With some of these antigens, particularly rubella, measles, and mumps vaccines, pregnancy is a contraindication to the vaccination. There is no convincing evidence of risk to the fetus from vaccination of pregnant women with inactivated viral vaccines or toxoids (such as diphtheria toxoid). (9:63)

271. **E.** Inactivated or killed vaccines do not multiply within the body; therefore, they pose no special problems for mothers who are breast-feeding or for their infants. Although live vaccines do multiply within the mother's body, most have not been demonstrated to be excreted in breast milk. In the few circumstances in which there could be transmission in breast milk (e.g., rubella), the virus usually does not infect the infant, and if it does the infection is well tolerated. (9:63)

272. **A.** To be acceptable for purposes of international travel, the yellow fever vaccine must be approved by the World Health Organization (WHO) and administered at a designated yellow fever vaccination center. Vaccination against typhus fever (epidemic louse-borne), plague, and meningococcal disease is not a requirement for entry into any country. (9:65)

273. **D.** Vaccination against typhoid fever is protective only against small infecting inocula. Periodic single reinforcing injections are desirable, usually at three- to five-year intervals. (6:384)

274. **B.** Toxoids produced from bacterial toxins artificially rendered harmless include diphtheria and tetanus vaccines. (6:116)

275. **C.** Infection does not confer effective immunity against tetanus and trachoma. One attack of smallpox usually confers lifelong immunity. (30:98)

276. **C.** The persistence of immunity following infection varies within wide limits. After a number of viral infections, such as measles and yellow fever, it is lifelong and does not depend on reinfection in order to be maintained. After streptococcal infection, gonorrhea, or treated syphilis, any immunity that may be developed is very transient. (37:77)

277. **E.** Although arthritis, pericarditis, and pneumonia occur, meningitis is the most common systemic manifestation of meningococcal disease. (37:191)

278. **E.** There is nothing characteristic about diphtheric skin lesions except their chronicity. Only rarely is a membrane seen at the base of a chronic ulcer. Rarely a patient with skin diphtheria may first present with a toxin-related complication of the infection. Other types of diphtheria include nasal diphtheria, aural diphtheria, diphtheritic conjunctivitis, mastoiditis, and labyrinthitis. (37:185)

CHAPTER THREE

Sexually Transmitted Diseases

Directions: Each of the questions or incomplete statements below is followed by five suggested answers or completions. Select the BEST answer in each case.

1. The primary lesion of syphilis (chancre) usually develops

   A. 21 days after birth in congenital syphilis
   B. less than one week after inoculation
   C. after an unknown period of incubation
   D. only after serologic tests for syphilis (STS) become reactive
   E. 10 to 90 days (average three weeks) after inoculation

2. Which of the following does not correspond with the description of a genital chancre?

   A. painful ulcer
   B. indurated base
   C. sharply demarcated borders
   D. usually solitary ulcer
   E. heals spontaneously in several weeks

3. Following effective treponemicidal therapy, the chancre becomes uninfectious after

   A. 24–48 hours
   B. seven days
   C. three weeks
   D. three months
   E. six months

4. About 70% of patients with secondary syphilis first present with

   A. ulcerated lesions of the mucous membranes
   B. "moth-eaten" alopecia
   C. lymph gland enlargement
   D. skin rash
   E. persistent hoarseness

5. Which of the following is not observed in the secondary stage of acquired syphilis?

   A. macular eruptions
   B. condyloma lata
   C. vesicular eruptions
   D. mucous patches
   E. "moth-eaten" alopecia

6. The most common site of syphilitic aneurysm is the

   A. abdominal aorta
   B. thoracic aorta
   C. left coronary artery
   D. right coronary artery
   E. brain arteries

7. The signs of early congenital syphilis may include all of the following except

   A. snuffles
   B. self-limited hemolytic anemia
   C. hepatosplenomegaly
   D. interstitial keratitis
   E. widespread lymphadenopathy

8. At present, which is the most sensitive (ability to be positive in persons having the disease) serologic test in all stages of syphilis?

    A. fluorescent treponemal antibody-absorption (FTA-ABS) test
    B. Kolmer test
    C. treponema pallidum immobilization test (TPI)
    D. venereal disease research laboratory (VDRL) test
    E. Kahn test

9. The treatment of syphilis in pregnancy

    A. does not require additional medication (penicillin)
    B. is contraindicated during the first trimester
    C. may cause retrolental fibroplasia
    D. for patients definitely known to be allergic to penicillin, tetracycline is the drug of choice
    E. requires higher doses of penicillin

10. If treatment of syphilis is begun after the eighteenth week of gestation

    A. penicillin is not the drug of choice
    B. only in exceptional cases is the baby cured
    C. mercury is the drug of choice
    D. it amounts to the treatment of the baby in utero
    E. erythromycin is the drug of choice

11. Among the untreated victims of syphilis, which of the following develops more frequently?

    A. arthritis
    B. insanity
    C. blindness
    D. cardiovascular disease
    E. deafness

12. In women, the primary infection of gonorrhea usually occurs in the

    A. urethra
    B. rectum
    C. throat
    D. vulva
    E. cervix

13. The most frequent cause of vulvovaginitis in childhood is

    A. gonorrhea
    B. moniliasis
    C. trichomoniasis
    D. foreign body
    E. *Chlamydia trachomatis* infections

14. Which of the following is the most common systemic (extragenital) complication of gonorrhea?

    A. myocarditis
    B. arthritis and tenosynovitis
    C. pericarditis
    D. meningitis
    E. endocarditis

15. Lymphogranuloma venereum is a sexually transmitted disease of

    A. fungal etiology
    B. rickettsial etiology
    C. chlamydial etiology
    D. treponemal etiology
    E. bacterial etiology

Directions: Each group of questions below consists of five lettered headings followed by a list of numbered words or phrases. For each numbered word or phrase select the one heading that is most closely related to it.

Questions 16 through 20

    A. *Treponema pallidum*
    B. *Neisseria gonorrhoeae*
    C. *Treponema pertenue*
    D. *Treponema refringens*
    E. *Treponema carateum*

16. endemic syphilis (Bejel)
17. rhagades
18. yaws (frambesia tropica, pian)
19. pinta
20. snuffles

Questions 21 through 25

A. Complement-fixation test
B. Gram's stain
C. Biopsy
D. Darkfield microscopy
E. Urine test

21. gonorrhea

22. secondary syphilis

23. lymphogranuloma venereum

24. yaws

25. pinta

Questions 26 through 30

A. Benzathine penicillin G: 2.4 million units total, intramuscular injections, at a single session
B. Benzathine penicillin G: 2.4 million units, intramuscular injections, once a week for three successive weeks (7.2 million units total)
C. Tetracycline HCl: 500 mg, by mouth, four times a day for 15 days
D. Erythromycin: 500 mg, by mouth, four times a day for 15 days
E. None of the above

26. chancre (positive darkfield); negative venereal disease research laboratory (VDRL) test

27. chancre (positive darkfield); reactive fluorescent treponemal antibody absorbed (FTA-ABS) test

28. women infected during late (multiple) pregnancy

29. coexistent chancre and secondary skin lesions

30. neurosyphilis

Questions 31 through 35

A. Tetracycline HCl: 500 mg, by mouth, four times a day for at least 2 weeks
B. Erythromycin: 500 mg, by mouth, four times a day, for a minimum of 10 days
C. Benzathine penicillin G units/kg, intramuscular inj single dose
D. Aqueous procaine penicillin units/kg, intramuscular injection, daily for a minimum of 10 days
E. Aqueous procaine penicillin G: 4.8 million units injected intramuscularly at two sites, with 1.0 g of probenecid by mouth

is the drug regimen of choice in

31. lymphogranuloma venereum

32. *Hemophilus ducreyi* infection (chancroid)

33. congenital syphilis (asymptomatic infants with normal cerebrospinal fluid)

34. congenital syphilis (symptomatic infants or asymptomatic infants with abnormal cerebrospinal fluid)

35. uncomplicated gonococcal infection in adults

Directions: Each set of lettered headings below is followed by a list of numbered words or phrases. For each numbered word or phrase select

A. if the item is associated with A only
B. if the item is associated with B only
C. if the item is associated with both A and B
D. if the item is associated with neither A nor B

Questions 36 through 40

A. Condyloma lata
B. Condyloma acuminatum (anogenital warts)
C. Both
D. Neither

36. caused by human papilloma virus

37. podophyllin is an effective therapy

38. moist, flat papules

39. these lesions are teeming with spirochetes

40. Serologic tests for syphilis are nonreactive

Questions 41 through 45

A. Acquired syphilis
B. Prenatal (congenital) syphilis
C. Both
D. Neither

41. neurosyphilis
42. cardiovascular involvement is extremely rare
43. chancre
44. bone lesions
45. syphilitic pemphigus

Questions 46 through 50

A. Nonvenereal (endemic) syphilis
B. Venereal syphilis
C. Both
D. Neither

46. the infectious stages of the disease are seen mainly in children
47. congenital transmission rarely if ever occurs
48. cardiovascular and neurologic involvement seems to be rare
49. mucous patches, condyloma lata
50. treponemes become blood-borne early in the infection

Questions 51 through 55

A. Pinta (carate)
B. Yaws (frambesia tropica, pian)
C. Both
D. Neither

51. the causative organism is of the same size, shape, and appearance of *Treponema pallidum*
52. provoke(s) identical antibody responses to those found in syphilis
53. clinical manifestations are confined to the skin
54. nonvenereal mode of transmission
55. penicillin is the treatment of choice

Questions 56 through 60

A. Chancre
B. Chancroid
C. Both
D. Neither

56. the incubation period is less than one week
57. soft, nonindurated, sharply circumscribed, and often painful ulcer
58. individual lesions are usually two to five in number
59. even without treatment, is usually self-limited
60. extragenital lesions have been noted

Questions 61 through 65

A. Lymphogranuloma venereum
B. Granuloma inguinale
C. Both
D. Neither

61. esthiomene, positive Frei skin test
62. rectal strictures are particularly common in women
63. has never been proved to be transmitted sexually
64. it is caused by *Calymmatobacterium granulomatis* (formerly termed *Donovania granulomatis*)
65. the incubation period is not accurately known

Directions: For each of the incomplete statements below, ONE or MORE of the completions given is correct. In each case select:

A. if only 1, 2, and 3 are correct
B. if only 1 and 3 are correct
C. if only 2 and 4 are correct
D. if only 4 is correct
E. if all are correct

66. In the secondary stage of syphilis
    1. a generalized or localized cutaneous eruption usually appears two weeks to six months (average six weeks) after inoculation
    2. lesions may appear before the chancre has healed
    3. lesions heal spontaneously after two to six weeks
    4. serologic tests for syphilis are uniformly negative

67. Gummata are sensitive reactions to the treponeme. They are found commonly in the
    1. bones
    2. heart
    3. skin
    4. nerves

68. Cardiovascular syphilis is often manifested by
    1. aortic aneurysm
    2. mitral stenosis
    3. aortic insufficiency
    4. aortic stenosis

69. Which of the following characterize(s) general paralysis of the insane (paresis)?
    1. symptoms are delayed on the average until 20 (or more) years after infection
    2. the memory is lost and judgment is impaired
    3. delusions of grandeur
    4. difficulty with speech

70. Which of the following characterize(s) locomotor ataxia (tabes dorsalis)?
    1. lancinating pains (lightning pains)
    2. bladder or bowel disturbances
    3. trophic joint changes (Charcot)
    4. loss of deep pain sensation associated with perforating soles or toes (mal perforans)

71. The mother was infected (syphilis) during the second trimester of pregnancy and received adequate treatment. The cord blood is reactive and
    1. the newborn should have a cerebrospinal fluid (CSF) examination before treatment
    2. three months after birth the baby will develop signs of early congenital syphilis
    3. the newborn should receive antisyphilitic treatment (penicillin) immediately
    4. the baby should be examined carefully at birth and at frequent intervals thereafter until nontreponemal serologic tests are negative

72. Syphilitic maternal infection occurred late in gestation. The infant was asymptomatic and seronegative at birth. The infant should be treated at birth if
    1. maternal treatment was inadequate
    2. maternal treatment was unknown
    3. maternal treatment was with drugs other than penicillin
    4. adequate followup cannot be ensured

73. Signs of late congenital syphilis include
    1. sabre skin
    2. saddle-nose configuration
    3. rhagades
    4. mulberry or Moon's molar

74. Which of the following statements about Hutchinson's teeth is (are) true?
    1. a sign of late congenital syphilis
    2. the permanent upper (occasionally the lower) central incisors develop a barrel-shaped and notched appearance and are smaller than normal
    3. the enamel is poorly formed, predisposing to cavities
    4. roentgen study of the unerupted teeth will allow the diagnosis to be made while the uninvolved deciduous teeth are still present

75. Darkfield examination may demonstrate the presence of *Treponema pallidum* in

    1. snuffles
    2. chancroid
    3. syphilitic mucous patches
    4. syphilitic gumma

76. "Specificity" of a test for syphilis refers to its ability to be nonreactive in the absence of the disease. Chronic biologic false-positive reactions have been associated with

    1. systemic lupus erythematosus
    2. lepromatous leprosy
    3. an elderly population
    4. measles

77. Which of the following have no place in the treatment of gonorrhea?

    1. tetracycline
    2. aqueous procaine penicillin G
    3. amoxicillin/ampicillin
    4. benzathine penicillin G

Answers and Explanations
Sexually Transmitted Diseases

1. **E.** Approximately three to four weeks (from as few as 10 days to as many as 90 days), after the treponeme has gained entrance into a new host, there develops at the portal of entry a primary lesion, the chancre. Serologic tests for syphilis are usually nonreactive when the chancre first appears but become reactive during the following one to four weeks. About half the patients seen during this stage will be seronegative. (59:22)

2. **A.** When free of other infectious agents, the chancre is typically painless. However, extragenital chancres may be painful. The lesion is usually an eroded papule that is decidedly firm and indurated. The surface may be crusted or ulcerated. The size varies from a few millimeters in diameter to 1 or 2 cm. The border surrounding the lesion is frequently raised and firm. The primary sore is usually a solitary ulcer. The lesion persists one to five weeks and then heals spontaneously. (59:22)

3. **A.** Following treatment, the primary or secondary syphilis chancres are free of active treponemes within 24–48 hours. If a bubo is present when treatment is begun, resolution of the gland may take several months. (4:84)

4. **D.** In practice, about 75% of patients with secondary syphilis first present with a skin rash, and about 50% will have a generalized enlargement of the lymph glands. There will be spots or sores on the mucous membranes in one third of cases. (4:75)

5. **C.** Vesicular eruptions are observed in congenital syphilis as opposed to acquired syphilis, in which vesicles are not seen. The skin lesions are bilaterally symmetrical and may be macular, papular, follicular, papulosquamous, or pustular. They are seldom pruritic and usually dry. Moist papules occur most frequently in the anogenital region (condylomata lata), but they may be seen on any body surface where moisture can accumulate between intertriginous surfaces (axillae or toe webs). Lesions of the mouth, throat, and cervix (mucous patches) frequently occur in secondary syphilis. "Moth-eaten" scalp alopecia, beginning in the occipital hair, is characteristic. (59:87)

6. **B.** Cardiovascular syphilis is usually caused by medial necrosis of the aorta. Saccular aneurysm of the thoracic aorta is prima facie evidence. Serologic tests for syphilis are usually reactive in cardiovascular syphilis. Syphilitic aortitis begins with perivascular inflammation of the vasa vasorum in the adventitia. Treponemas subsequently invade the media via the lymphatics, producing medial inflammation and destruction. Aneurysm caused by atherosclerosis usually affects the abdominal aorta. (59:82)

7. **D.** The early stage of congenital syphilis is characterized by the appearance of signs and symptoms before the age of two years. The earlier the onset in the first weeks of life, usually the poorer the prognosis. Interstitial keratitis usually appears near puberty and eventually becomes bilateral. The cornea develops a ground-glass appearance, with vascularization of the adjacent sclera. The mucous membranes of the nose and pharynx are frequently involved, producing a heavy mucoid discharge referred to as "the snuffles." Most cases have a hemolytic anemia that is self-limited. Hepatosplenomegaly is frequently present (two thirds of cases) and may be associated with a low-grade icterus. There may be a widespread lymphadenopathy. (59:89)

8. **A.** The standard treponemal test in the United States is the manual fluorescent treponemal antibody-absorption (FTA-ABS) test, which is based on indirect immunofluorescence testing techniques. (16:1709)

9. **A.** For patients at all stages of pregnancy who are

not allergic to penicillin, penicillin should be used in dosage schedules appropriate for the stage of syphilis as recommended for the treatment of nonpregnant patients. Retrolental fibroplasia can be produced by long exposure of premature infants to high concentrations of oxygen. Tetracycline is not recommended in pregnant women because of potential adverse effects on the fetus. Tetracycline should not be given to children less than eight years of age. For patients at all stages of pregnancy who have documented allergy to penicillin, if compliance and serologic followup can be assured, administer erythromycin in dosage schedules appropriate for the stage of syphilis as recommended for treatment of nonpregnant patients. Infants born to mothers treated with erythromycin for early syphilis during pregnancy should be treated with penicillin. (11:52S)

10. **D.** Adequate treatment of the mother before the eighteenth week of pregnancy prevents infection of the fetus. Because penicillin will cross the placenta in adequate amounts, treatment of the mother after the eighteenth week of pregnancy will usually bring about in utero cure but may not prevent bone or joint involvement, neural deafness, or interstitial keratitis in the newborn. (59:86)

11. **D.** Latent disease follows secondary syphilis for life in an asymptomatic form in 60–70% of patients, or progresses to neurosyphilis (6.5%), cardiovascular disease (9.6%), or late benign gummata (16%). (16:1683)

12. **E.** The cervix is the site most commonly infected (about 90% of cases). The urethra is the next most common site at 75%; the rectum at 40%; the throat at 6% of cases. (4:31)

13. **D.** Typical foreign bodies include items like beans, buttons, paper clips, and toilet paper. (4:60)

14. **B.** Arthritis, because of joint involvement secondary to bacteremia, is the most common complication of gonorrhea and, if untreated, may lead to ankylosis of the joint. The heart may be involved in a gonococcal myocarditis, pericarditis, or endocarditis. Meningitis is quite rare and is interesting because of the similarity between gonococcus and meningococcus. (4:37)

15. **C.** Lymphogranuloma venereum's causative agent is a member of the chlamydia group. (4:92)

16. **A.** *Treponema pallidum,* a spirochete, is the etiologic agent of nonvenereal syphilis (Bejel). (16:1726)

17. **A.** Rhagades is a sign of late congenital syphilis. (59:91)

18. **C.** *Treponema pertenue,* a spirochete, is the etiologic agent of yaws. (4:95)

19. **E.** *Treponema carateum,* a spirochete, is the etiologic agent of pinta (carate). (4:96)

20. **A.** The snuffles is a sign of early congenital syphilis. (59:87)

21. **B.** Definitive diagnosis of gonorrhea depends upon identification of the organisms by Gram's stain. (16:1747)

22. **D.** Darkfield examination may be helpful in confirming the diagnosis of secondary syphilis. (16:1693)

23. **A.** The diagnosis of LV is made on the basis of clinical findings and the complement-fixation test. (16:1740)

24. **D.** Diagnosis of yaws is by darkfield examination and STS. (16:1728)

25. **D.** Diagnosis of pinta is made by demonstrating *Treponema carateum* from early skin lesions and a reactive STS. (16:1729)

26. **A.** Early syphilis (primary, secondary, latent syphilis of less than one year's duration) should be treated with benzathine penicillin G: 2.4 million units total, IM, at a single session. Patients who are allergic to penicillin should be treated with tetracycline HCl: 500 mg, by mouth, four times daily for 15 days. (11:50S)

27. **A.** Early syphilis treatment. (11:50S)

28. **A.** Early syphilis treatment. (11:50S)

29. **A.** Early syphilis treatment. (11:50S)

30. **B.** Published studies show that a total dose of 6 to 9 million units of penicillin G over a three- to four-week period results in satisfactory clinical response in approximately 90% of patients with neurosyphilis. This information must be considered along with the observation that regimens employing benzathine penicillin or procaine penicillin in doses under 2.4 million units daily do not consistently provide treponemicidal levels of penicillin in cerebrospinal fluid (CSF), and with the knowledge that several case reports show the failure of such regimens to cure neurosyphilis. (11:51S)

31. **A.** The following drugs are active against LGV serotypes in vitro but have not been evaluated extensively in culture-confirmed cases: doxycycline, erythromycin, and sulfa methoxazole. Fluctuant lymph nodes should be aspirated as needed through

healthy adjacent normal skin. Incision and drainage or excision of nodes will delay healing and are contraindicated. Late sequelae such as stricture and/or fistula may require surgical intervention. (11:54S)

32. **B.** Infection with *Hemophilus ducreyi* should be treated with erythromycin or trimethoprim/sulfamethoxazole: double-strength tablet (160/800 mg) by mouth, twice a day. Therapy should be continued for a minimum of 10 days and until ulcers and/or lymph nodes have healed. Fluctuant lymph nodes should be aspirated through healthy adjacent normal skin. Incision and drainage or excision of nodes will delay healing and are contraindicated. Apply compresses to ulcers to remove necrotic material. (11:54S)

33. **C.** Only penicillin regimens are recommended for neonatal congenital syphilis. (11:53S)

34. **D.** If neurosyphilis cannot be excluded, the aqueous crystalline or procaine penicillin regimen is recommended. (11:53S)

35. **E.** The advantage of this regimen in the treatment of gonorrhea is that it is a single-dose therapy. Disadvantages: injection; possible procaine reaction; possible penicillin anaphylaxis; ineffective against chlamydial infections. (11:37S)

36. **B.** Condyloma acuminatum is caused by an epidermotropic DNA virus—human papilloma virus (HPV), a member of the papova group. (16:1631)

37. **B.** Anogenital warts often respond to 25% podophyllum in a tincture. (16:1672)

38. **A.** Condyloma lata are moist, flat papules. Condyloma acuminatum is usually not flat but more sessile, pedunculated, or filiform. (16:1780)

39. **A.** These lesions (condyloma lata) are teeming with spirochetes. They are quite infectious. (16:1688)

40. **B.** The serologic tests for syphilis are nonreactive in condyloma acuminatum. (16:1690)

41. **C.** Neurosyphilis occurs in one-third to one-half of patients with prenatal syphilis. (59:91)

42. **B.** Cardiovascular involvement is extremely rare. (59:91)

43. **A.** Since spirochetemia is the source of infection, from mother to fetus, in utero, the "primary" stage of acquired syphilis chancre is bypassed. (16:1702)

44. **C.** In acquired syphilis bone lesions are usually marked by periostitis with associated new bone formation or by gummatous osteitis with bone destruction. The cardinal signs are pain, swelling, and bony tumor. The most common sites are the cranial bones, the tibia, and the clavicle. In early congenital syphilis, osteochondritis of the long bones occurs. Dactylitis results from involvement of the phalanges. In late congenital syphilis the process may be sclerotic (saber shin), with frontal bossing, or it may be lytic (gummatous) and produce destruction, most frequently of the nasal septum (the saddle nose configuration) or the hard palate. Perforation of the palate is very suggestive of congenital syphilis. Any part of the skeletal system may be involved. (59:85)

45. **B.** Although rare, bullous lesions of early syphilis (syphilitic pemphigus) are characteristic of the disease. (16:1702)

46. **A.** Most infections are acquired in childhood, with subsequent diminished susceptibility to sexually transmitted treponematosis in adult life. The disease is found in communities with low socio-economic status. (62:148)

47. **A.** Untreated females are generally noninfectious when the fertile years are reached; conversely, an infant infected from another source may superinfect the parent. (62:148)

48. **A.** Cardiovascular and neurologic involvement seems to be rare in endemic syphilis. (16:1727)

49. **C.** Lesions are often clinically identical. (62:148)

50. **C.** All the treponemes of these diseases almost certainly become blood-borne early in the infection. (35:403)

51. **C.** The causative organisms of the nonvenereal treponematoses are morphologically identical. (16:1725)

52. **C.** Reactive serologic tests. (4:94)

53. **A.** The destructive lesions seen in yaws do not occur in pinta, and bone lesions seldom cause trouble. (4:96)

54. **C.** Both are nonvenereally transmitted. (16:1725)

55. **C.** Mass treatment with penicillin or other antibiotics is required. (4:96)

56. **B.** The incubation period of chancroid is generally accepted as being three to five days. (16:1736)

57. **B.** In contrast to syphilis, the ulcers of chancroid are usually tender and often painful. (16:1736)

58. **B.** Individual lesions are usually two to five in number in chancroid. The chancre is usually a single lesion. (16:1684)

59. **C.** Even without treatment, the chancroid is usually self-limited. Healing of the chancre takes place over three to six weeks, even without treatment, and leaves a thin atrophic scar. (16:1737)

60. **C.** Extragenital chancroids have been noted within the mouth or on the umbilicus, lips, breasts, and conjunctivae. Extragenital chancres may occur anywhere, but have been most commonly observed in the anus or rectum, mouth, lips, tongue, tonsils, fingers, toes, umbilicus, breasts, and eyelids. (16:1736)

61. **A.** Because lymphogranuloma venereum affects the lymph channels and glands, there is disruption of the normal fluid drainage from the genital area. The result is the development of chronic lymphatic edema, and eventually elephantiasis. This complication causes a gross swelling of the perineum called esthiomene. (4:93)

62. **A.** Because of the close proximity of the vagina to the rectum, women are more prone to suffer the so-called "ano-rectal syndrome." (4:93)

63. **B.** It is possible that transmission of GI is by sexual contact, although this has not yet been definitely proved. Sexual consorts of patients with the disease are often unaffected. (4:93)

64. **B.** It has not been possible to pass the disease (GI) on to animals or to human volunteers by inoculation of the organism. (4:94)

65. **B.** The incubation period of granuloma inguinale is not accurately known but may be as much as two months. The incubation period of lymphogranuloma venereum is usually between one and two weeks, although longer periods have been reported. (4:94)

66. **A.** In about 30% of patients the primary chancre is found to be present when secondary lesions appear. Practically every case of secondary syphilis shows strongly positive reactions. (4:75)

67. **E.** The basic pathologic lesion in tertiary syphilis is a chronic granuloma known as gumma. (62:61)

68. **B.** The essential signs of cardiovascular syphilis are those of aortic insufficiency or saccular aneurysm of the thoracic aorta. Saccular aneurysm of the thoracic aorta is prima facie evidence of cardiovascular syphilis. Aortic insufficiency with no other valvular lesions in a person of middle age with a reactive serologic test should be considered cardiovascular syphilis until proved otherwise. (59:82)

69. **E.** Signs and symptoms of paresis are always indicative of widespread parenchymatous damage. Personality changes range from minor to frankly psychotic. Frequently there are focal neurologic signs. (4:80)

70. **E.** Prime signs and symptoms of tabes dorsalis are those of posterior column degeneration. (59:77)

71. **D.** If the mother has received adequate penicillin treatment during pregnancy, the risk to the infant is minimal. All children showing reactive serologic tests must be followed with serial serologic tests. A falling titer represents catabolic loss of passively transferred reagin; rising titers indicate active infection requiring treatment. (59:107)

72. **E.** Infected infants are frequently asymptomatic at birth and may be seronegative if the maternal infection occurred late in gestation. Infants should be treated at birth if maternal treatment was inadequate, unknown, or with drugs other than penicillin, or if inadequate followup of the infant cannot be ensured. (11:52S)

73. **E.** Sabre shin is a result of periostitis of the anterior and middle portion of the tibia, with a resultant thickening and bowing. Saddle nose is the end result of syphilitic rhinitis. Rhagades are the end result of linear fissures or ulcers or early prenatal disease. In mulberry or Moon's molar the first lower molar may show maldevelopment of the cusps. All the molars may be affected. (16:1704)

74. **E.** Due to the poor development of the middle denticle, the permanent upper (occasionally the lower) central incisors develop a barrel-shaped and notched appearance and are smaller than normal, causing the teeth to be more widely spaced. (59:90)

75. **B.** Darkfield is negative in chancroid. *Treponema pallidum* is only rarely found in gummatous lesions. (59:39)

76. **A.** Biologic false-positive (BFP) reactors for the reaginic tests are defined as patients in whom one or more of these tests (VDRL, Kahn, Wasserman, etc.) are repeatedly positive, but in whom tests for antitreponemal antibody (FTA and/or TPI test) are negative. Acute positivity reverts to negativity within six months of the first positive finding, and chronic reactors are those in whom positivity persists for six months or longer. Measles is a transient reactor. (16:1707)

77. **D.** Although long-acting forms of penicillin (such as benzathine penicillin G) are effective in the treatment of syphilis, they have no place in the treatment of gonorrhea. Oral penicillin preparations such as penicillin V are not recommended for the treatment of gonococcal infection. (11:39S)

CHAPTER FOUR

Nutrition and Deficiency Diseases

Directions: Each of the questions or incomplete statements below is followed by five suggested answers or completions. Select the BEST answer in each case.

1. Particularly common in underdeveloped areas of the world is

    A. carbohydrate deficiency
    B. protein–calorie deficiency
    C. mineral deficiency
    D. fat-soluble vitamin deficiency
    E. water-soluble vitamin deficiency

2. Which of the following aspects of nutrition requires considerable attention in the United States?

    A. scurvy
    B. obesity
    C. beriberi
    D. pellagra
    E. ricketts

3. The daily recommended calorie intake for an average-sized, physically active 22-year-old man weighing 70 kilos is

    A. 1,300
    B. 1,700
    C. 2,400
    D. 2,600
    E. 2,900

4. Which of the following is characterized by changes in the color of the hair, skin lesions, diarrhea, edema, and enlarged liver?

    A. dermatomyositis
    B. pellagra
    C. kwashiorkor
    D. acrodynia
    E. vitiligo

5. All of the following are fat- or oil-soluble vitamins *except*

    A. vitamin A
    B. vitamin C
    C. vitamin D
    D. vitamin E
    E. vitamin K

6. Massive doses of which of the following may cause hepatosplenomegaly, hypoplastic anemia, leukopenia, precocious skeletal development, clubbing of the fingers, and coarse, sparse hair?

    A. vitamin A
    B. vitamin D
    C. vitamin K
    D. vitamin E
    E. cyanocobalamin

7. Which of the following has been dramatically effective in the treatment of Wernicke's syndrome (cerebral beriberi)?

    A. ascorbic acid

67

B. thiamine
C. vitamin D
D. vitamin A
E. antihistaminics

8. "Burning feet syndrome" is due to
   A. panthothenic acid deficiency
   B. iron deficiency
   C. calcium deficiency
   D. iodine deficiency
   E. pyridoxine (vitamin B₆) deficiency

9. A major public health problem throughout the world is
   A. hemolytic anemia (acquired)
   B. thalassemia
   C. iron-deficiency anemia
   D. nutritional megaloblastic anemia
   E. malabsorption megaloblastic anemia

Directions: Each group of questions below consists of five lettered headings followed by a list of numbered words or phrases. For each numbered word or phrase select the one heading that is most closely related to it.

Questions 10 through 14

   A. Vitamin A (retinol)
   B. Vitamin D (calciferol)
   C. Vitamin C (ascorbic acid)
   D. Vitamin K
   E. Vitamin B₆ (pyridoxine)

10. hypocalcemia, hypophosphatemia, rickets in infants and children, osteomalacia in adults

11. essential for growth and bone development in children, for vision (particularly in dim light), and for integrity of mucosal and epithelial surfaces

12. acts as a reducing agent and antioxidant, subperiosteal hemorrhages, ecchymoses

13. hypoprothrombinemia; hemorrhagic disease of the newborn

14. inadequate utilization has been implicated in a number of conditions that appear to be genetically determined, indicated to prevent or treat peripheral neuritis caused by isoniazid

Questions 15 through 19

   A. Vitamin E (alpha tocopherol)
   B. Vitamin B₁ (thiamine)
   C. niacin
   D. vitamin B₁₂
   E. vitamin B₅ (pantothenic acid)

15. essential nutrient that protects polyunsaturated fatty acids from oxidative deterioration

16. an essential coenzyme for carbohydrate metabolism; essential for nerve cell and heart tissue function

17. deficiency may be associated with carcinoid syndrome (deviation of precursor tryptophan for conversion by tumor to serotonin)

18. a generic term for several cobalt-containing compounds; as a component of various coenzymes, it is important in the synthesis of nucleic acid

19. as a precursor of coenzyme A, it is essential in the intermediary metabolism of fats, carbohydrates, and proteins

Questions 20 through 24

   A. Ascorbic acid (vitamin C) deficiency
   B. Vitamin B₁ (thiamine) deficiency
   C. Vitamin B₂ (riboflavin) deficiency
   D. Vitamin B₃ (niacin) deficiency
   E. Vitamin D (calciferol) deficiency

20. neurasthenia, loss of attention, irritability, vague fears, emotional disturbance

21. "angular stomatitis"; "cheilosis"

22. failure to form and maintain intercellular substance; the child does not voluntarily move the extremities because of pain

23. achlorhydria; the tongue loses its papillae and becomes bright red and sore

24. bowed legs, flat feet, rachitic rosary, pigeon breast

Directions: Each set of lettered headings below is followed by a list of numbered words or phrases. For each numbered word or phrase select

  A. if the item is associated with A only
  B. if the item is associated with B only
  C. if the item is associated with both A and B
  D. if the item is associated with neither A nor B

Questions 25 through 29

  A. Folic acid
  B. Vitamin B$_{12}$
  C. Both
  D. Neither

25. megaloblastic anemia

26. deficiency causes lesions in the spinal cord and optic nerve

27. has found its greatest usefulness in treatment of the macrocytic anemia of pregnancy

28. highly effective in relieving the combined system disease of pernicious anemia

29. absorption may be interfered with by the fish tapeworm (Dibothriocephalus latus)

Directions: For each of the incomplete statements below, ONE or MORE of the completions given is correct. In each case select:

  A. if only 1, 2, and 3 are correct
  B. if only 1 and 3 are correct
  C. if only 2 and 4 are correct
  D. if only 4 is correct
  E. if all are correct

30. Clinical signs of vitamin A deficiency include
  1. follicular hyperkeratosis
  2. xerophthalmia
  3. keratomalacia
  4. nyctalopia

31. Bitot's spots
  1. occur only in situations in which malnutrition exists or has existed recently
  2. are pathognomonic in measles

Nutrition and Deficiency

  3. may reflect a milder f...
     xerosis of the conjur...
  4. improve with antihi...

32. Symptoms of poisoning may resu... cessive intake of
  1. vitamin A
  2. vitamin B
  3. vitamin D
  4. vitamin C

33. Clinical signs of nicotinamide deficiency include
  1. dermatitis
  2. dementia
  3. diarrhea
  4. flushing reaction

34. Thiamine deficiency in human beings may be associated with
  1. foot drop
  2. sensory neuropathy of the peripheral type, with glove and stocking anesthesia
  3. enlargement of the heart
  4. atony and dilatation of the bowel

35. Scrotal dermatitis is due to
  1. lack of calcium
  2. lack of ascorbic acid
  3. lack of iodine
  4. lack of riboflavin

36. Spongy, bleeding gums may be an expression of
  1. lack of vitamin C
  2. non-nutritional periodontal disease
  3. lymphoma
  4. dilantin toxicity

37. Glossitis may be due to a lack of
  1. niacin
  2. iron tryptophan
  3. vitamin B$_{12}$
  4. riboflavin

Glossitis areata exfoliativa (geographic tongue)

1. is characterized by asymptomatic, circinate patches of atrophic erythematous mucosa
2. is of particular importance in the diagnosis of lead poisoning
3. the cause and pathogenesis are unknown
4. is always associated with hypersensitivity to light

Answers and Explanations
Nutrition and Deficiency Diseases

1. **B.** Protein–calorie malnutrition is easily the most important nutrition problem of the whole world, though deficiencies due to vitamins A, B, and D are also quite common. (30:241)

2. **B.** Obesity is perhaps the most prevalent form of malnutrition in the United States and other industrialized countries. (37:1575)

3. **E.** The committee on foods and nutrition of the National Research Council recommends a 2,900 calorie intake for an average sized, physically active 22-year-old man, and 2,100 calories for an active woman of the same age but of lesser weight. (37:1473)

4. **C.** The principal signs of kwashiorkor are changes in the color and texture of the hair; desquamating, pigmented, superficially ulcerated skin lesions that frequently resemble those of pellagra; diarrhea; an enlarged liver; and severe edema. (37:1473)

5. **B.** In general, vitamins may be water-soluble, such as the B vitamins and vitamin C, or fat-soluble, as is the case with vitamins A and D. (20:163)

6. **A.** Most symptoms, but not hepatomegaly and abnormal bone growth, clear with discontinuation of the vitamin. (37:1483)

7. **B.** Wernicke's encephalopathy with its external rectus palsy, together with cerebral symptoms, is attributable to thiamine deficiency. (35:584)

8. **A.** "Burning feet" have been the only or outstanding complaint. (35:539)

9. **C.** Iron deficiency is a major health problem all over the world, especially in women during their reproductive years (particularly during pregnancy) and in infants. (35:678)

10. **B.** (35:824)

11. **A.** (35:822)

12. **C.** (35:827)

13. **D.** (35:827)

14. **E.** (35:831)

15. **A.** (35:825)

16. **B.** (35:832)

17. **C.** (35:830)

18. **D.** (35:833)

19. **E.** (35:830)

20. **B.** These are the earliest symptoms of beriberi, due to vitamin B_1 deficiency. (37:1478)

21. **C.** The symptoms that may be associated with riboflavin deficiency can be classified as oral, dermal, and ocular. (37:1479)

22. **A.** Vitamin C deficiency (scurvy). (37:1480)

23. **D.** Niacin deficiency (pellagra). (37:1480)

24. **E.** Vitamin D deficiency (rickets). (37:1477)

25. **C.** Since both folic acid and vitamin B_{12} are essential cofactors for DNA synthesis, a deficiency of either causes defective cell division, which inhibits normal reproduction of proliferating cells, including hematopoietic cells. (2:1060)

26. **B.** Deficiency of vitamin B_{12} may be associated with subacute combined degeneration of the spinal cord. (2:833)

27. **A.** Folic acid alleviates the megaloblastic anemias that occur during pregnancy. (2:1063)

28. **B.** Prompt parenteral administration of vitamin B$_{12}$ prevents progression of neurologic damage. (2:833)

29. **B.** The fish tapeworm is the largest tapeworm found in man and is known to reach up to 30 feet. The worm is of particular interest because it causes a type of pernicious anemia through competition for vitamin B$_{12}$ in the human gut. (25:63)

30. **E.** Vitamin A deficiency: Follicular hyperkeratosis may appear first on the extensor surface of the thighs and lateral surface of the forearms. Eye lesions result from lacrimal gland changes that cause drying and thickening of the conjunctiva (xerophthalmia). As the disease progresses to keratomalacia (dryness with perforation and ulceration of the cornea), the erosion may enlarge rapidly, with protrusion and eventual prolapse of the iris, resulting in total blindness. One of the common symptoms is night blindness (nictalopia). (37:1477)

31. **B.** It is possible that the localized lesions, known as Bitot's spots, reflect a milder form of nutritional xerosis of the conjunctiva of this type, restricted to the most exposed area of the bulb. What is certain is that Bitot's spots occur only in situations in which malnutrition exists or has existed recently. If nutritional xerosis of the cornea is treated (vitamin A) early, the condition can be reversed and the sight saved. (35:582)

32. **B.** Hypervitaminosis A and D. (37:1483)

33. **A.** The cardinal signs of pellagra constitute the well-known triad of diarrhea, dermatitis, and dementia. Therapeutic doses of niacin may cause flushing reactions. (35:535)

34. **E.** The symptoms of thiamine deficiency may be classified as neurologic, cardiac, and gastrointestinal. (37:1478)

35. **D.** Scrotal dermatitis, an eczematous condition of the scrotum, is due to ariboflavinosis. (35:538)

36. **E.** Spongy, bleeding gums may be an expression of lack of vitamin C, periodontal disease due to poor oral hygiene, lack of dental care, lymphoma, or toxicity from dilantin. (49:7)

37. **E.** The tongue is beefy red, painful, and may be fissured. Symptoms of hypersensitivity, burning, and changes in taste sensation almost always occur. (49:7)

38. **B.** The atrophy is due to loss of filiform papillae. The lesions have been thought to be due to vitamin deficiency, emotional stress, etc. (16:870)

CHAPTER FIVE

Occupational Diseases of the Skin

Directions: Each of the questions or incomplete statements below is followed by five suggested answers or completions. Select the BEST answer in each case.

1. Generalized pruritus occurs, often as the presenting symptom, in *(usually normal looking skin)*

   A. Hodgkin's disease
   B. mycosis fungoides
   C. leukemia
   D. multiple myeloma
   E. all of the above

2. Which of the following statements concerning occupational dermatosis (a pathologic condition of the skin for which job exposure can be a direct cause or contributory factor), is (are) true?

   A. lack of cleanliness is probably the most common cause of dermatitis
   B. areas of thickened skin reduce the chance of contact allergy
   C. fair-skinned individuals working outdoors are at risk of skin damage from sunlight
   D. many of the individuals most frequently affected with acute skin lesions are young
   E. all of the above

3. Which of the following are the most frequent of the occupational diseases?

   A. ear conditions
   B. respiratory conditions
   C. eye conditions
   D. skin conditions
   E. systemic effects of toxic materials

4. Most occupational skin diseases are caused by

   A. biologic agents
   B. physical agents
   C. mechanical agents
   D. chemical agents
   E. unspecified agents

5. Which of the following measures can be instituted to help prevent occupational skin diseases?

   A. pre-use testing and evaluation
   B. engineering and industrial hygiene
   C. personal hygiene
   D. personal protective clothing
   E. all of the above

6. Primary lesions that may be observed in occupational dermatoses include

   A. macules
   B. papules
   C. nodules
   D. vesicles
   E. all of the above

73

7. Which of the following is the most common form of occupational dermatoses?

   A. pigmentary disturbances
   B. pilosebaceous reactions
   C. neoplasms
   D. contact dermatitis
   E. vascular changes

8. On the basis of the incidence of occupational skin diseases, which of the following is the industry with highest risk?

   A. leather tanning and finishing
   B. poultry dressing
   C. adhesives and sealants
   D. boat building and repairing
   E. fresh or frozen packaged fish

9. Contact epilating folliculitis is an occupational disease observed among

   A. sugar cane workers
   B. road workers
   C. farmers
   D. fishermen
   E. telephone linemen

10. Which of the following metals produces the greatest number of clinically significant patch-test reactions?

    A. gold
    B. sodium
    C. potassium
    D. mercury
    E. nickel

11. All of the following statements concerning lichen planus are true except

    A. it may involve the mucous membranes but tends to spare the face, palms, and soles
    B. it is characterized by papules that are flat-topped, polygonal, violaceous, and surmounted by thin, silvery scale
    C. severe dystrophy of the nails may be observed
    D. the most reliable aid to diagnosis is examination of scrapings from lesions
    E. occasionally affects the scalp and causes permanent scarring alopecia

12. Pityriasis rubra pilaris is characterized by all of the following except

    A. hyperkeratotic palmar lesions
    B. acuminate follicular papules on the dorsa of fingers
    C. scaling dermatitis with islands of normal skin
    D. low serum levels of vitamin A have been reported
    E. ultraviolet-light treatment, as used for psoriasis, is the most successful treatment

13. "Herald patch" commonly antedates the generalized eruption by several days or weeks in

    A. measles
    B. pityriasis rosea
    C. syphilis
    D. drug reactions
    E. acute psoriasis

14. Pityriasis rosea is characterized by all of the following except

    A. the cause and method of transmission are unknown
    B. the trunk lesions tend to have their long axis parallel to the ribs, giving a "Christmas tree" distribution to the lesions
    C. the patient usually experiences only minimal pruritus
    D. recurrences are usual
    E. generally remits spontaneously in four to eight weeks

15. Reiter's syndrome is characterized by all of the following except

    A. arthritis, urethritis, and conjunctivitis
    B. hyperkeratotic, erosive, and psoriasiform lesions
    C. children are most commonly affected
    D. no causative organism has yet been identified
    E. there is no specific laboratory test for the diagnosis of this condition

16. Unusual reactivity to the sun is not observed in

    A. systemic lupus erythematosus
    B. porphyria cutanea tarda

C. pellagra
D. albinism
E. xanthomata

17. Which statement about psoriasis is *incorrect*?
    A. genetic and environmental factors contribute to the clinical disease
    B. the sexes are equally affected and the onset may be at any age
    C. it is commoner in southern climates
    D. arthritis (usually polyarticular with a predilection for the small joints of hands and feet) is common
    E. plaques are topped by white or silvery scales

18. Which of the following is *not* a characteristic of atopic dermatitis?
    A. there is a marked familial tendency to allergic diseases
    B. the flexures are commonly attacked (adult type)
    C. striking seasonal variation is seen in some patients with deterioration in either very warm or very cold climates
    D. lesions are not particularly itchy
    E. there is typical facial pallor and infraorbital darkening

19. Nummular eczematous dermatitis is characterized by all of the following *except*
    A. coin-shaped lesions often distributed on the legs, upper extremities, and the trunk
    B. pruritus is variable and can be absent
    C. the lesions are: papules, vesicles, crusts
    D. one of the most frequent occupational dermatoses
    E. the cause is unknown

20. Seborrheic dermatitis is characterized by all of the following *except*
    A. involves the scalp, central face, presternal and crural areas
    B. commonly asymptomatic
    C. the course is chronic, with recurrences and remissions
    D. unknown etiology
    E. the most common of all skin conditions

21. Which of the following statements concerning stasis dermatitis is correct?
    A. signs of venous insufficiency (varicosities, pigmentation, ulcers)
    B. the lesions are most common over the region of the medial malleolus
    C. pruritus may be severe
    D. treatment of the underlying venous insufficiency is the most important form of therapy
    E. all of the above

22. Which of the following statements concerning furuncles is *incorrect*?
    A. an acute painful infection of a hair follicle
    B. the resulting permanent scar is often dense and readily evident
    C. sites commonly affected are the neck, face, axillae, and buttocks
    D. may be associated with systemic host factors
    E. the cause is usually streptococci

23. Which of the following entities is no longer considered related to tuberculosis?
    A. erythema induratum
    B. tuberculous chancre
    C. lupus vulgaris
    D. papulo necrotic tuberculid
    E. lupus miliaris disseminatus faciei

24. All of the following are diseases caused by viruses *except*
    A. herpes simplex
    B. dermatitis herpetiformis
    C. warts
    D. Kaposi's varicelliform eruption
    E. molluscum contagiosum

25. Which of the following statements concerning warts is *incorrect*?
    A. the peak incidence occurs during the second decade of life
    B. trauma plays some factor in inoculation
    C. fingers are the chief site of common warts (verruga vulgaris)

D. some individuals are more susceptible than others
E. anogenital warts (condylomata acuminata) are syphilitic lesions

26. Which of the following does *not* correspond with the description of molluscum contagiosum?
    A. this disorder is not uncommon in beauty specialists
    B. involves clusters of pearly papules that become umbilicated as they grow
    C. the etiologic agent is both autoinoculable and contagious
    D. biopsy is always required for diagnosis
    E. most cases resolve spontaneously

27. All of the following are fungal infections *except*
    A. thrush
    B. kerion
    C. tinea corporis (ringworm)
    D. tinea pedia (athlete's foot)
    E. erythrasma

28. The clinical features of candidiasis (moniliasis) include
    A. onychia and paronychia
    B. vaginitis
    C. intraoral thrush
    D. superficial glossitis
    E. all of the above

29. Which of the following conditions may predispose to candida infection?
    A. obesity
    B. alcoholism
    C. diabetes
    D. hyperhidrosis
    E. all of the above

30. Which of the following statements concerning tinea circinata (tinea corporis) is *incorrect*?
    A. practically all species of tricophyton and microsporum are capable of involving any area of smooth skin
    B. the diagnosis is made by microscopy, and culture when necessary
    C. Wood's light is positive in some cases when the scalp is involved
    D. it is an occupational disease among farmers
    E. corticosteroid ointment is the treatment of choice

31. Which of the following statements concerning pityriasis versicolor (tinea versicolor) is *incorrect*?
    A. the lesions are mainly on the trunk and proximal part of the limbs
    B. itching and burning sensations are usual and severe
    C. selenium sulphide suspension is a useful preparation
    D. the lesions are macular and fawn-colored or café-au-lait
    E. it is a fungal infection

32. Diagnosis of pityriasis versicolor (tinea versicolor) is made by
    A. occupational history
    B. serologic tests
    C. histologic examination
    D. intradermal skin test
    E. finding fungus in scales

33. Scabies is characterized by all of the following *except*
    A. the mites (Sarcoptes scabiei) live in cutaneous burrows several millimeters to a few centimeters in length
    B. itching is less severe at night
    C. frequent sites of itching are the interdigital skin and genital area
    D. the back is seldom involved, and the head is almost always exempt, except in infants
    E. all household and other close contacts of confirmed cases of scabies should be treated at the same time as the patient

34. Which of the following statements concerning pediculosis corporis is *incorrect*?
    A. the body louse resides in, and lays eggs near, the seams of the clothing

B. pruritus is a prominent symptom
C. postinflammatory hyperpigmentation may develop
D. endemic or murine typhus is caused by *Rickettsia mooseri*, which is transmitted to humans by *Pediculus humanus*
E. Parallel linear excoriations in the interscapular region are almost pathognomonic

35. Which of the following corresponds with the description of folliculitis barbae?
    A. a chronic staphylococcal infection of the hair follicles of the beard and moustache areas
    B. the lesions are follicular and consist of pustules and crusts
    C. blepharitis is a common accompaniment
    D. itching and pain may be present
    E. all of the above

36. Which of the following does *not* correspond with the description of impetigo vulgari?
    A. the organisms commonly identified are *Staphylococcus aureus* and group A streptococci
    B. the lesions are covered with a heavy honey-colored crust
    C. the causative organism can spread quickly, particularly among children
    D. generally found on exposed areas
    E. usually associated with diabetes mellitus

37. Which of the following statements concerning systemic lupus erythematosus is *incorrect*?
    A. skin lesions are always present
    B. any organ in the body may be affected
    C. sunlight and offensive drugs must be avoided
    D. women are more often affected than men
    E. the treatment is usually based on systemic corticosteroids

38. Concerning chronic lupus erythematosus, which of the following statements is *incorrect*?

    A. lesions in the scalp destroy the hair bulbs, leaving a permanent scarring alopecia
    B. antinuclear factor is found in about 20% of cases
    C. lesions are often most pronounced on the upper cheeks
    D. scaly discoid lesions are found with the unique plugging of the follicles
    E. antibiotics are the drugs of choice

39. Which of the following statements concerning dermatomyositis is *incorrect*?
    A. chelating agents are the treatment of choice
    B. edema and a purplish-red periorbital discoloration are most marked over the upper lids (heliotrope erythema)
    C. subcutaneous calcium deposits may be extruded
    D. muscle biopsy is the most definite diagnostic test
    E. no infectious agent has been isolated in tissues

40. Associated with erythema nodosum is (are)
    A. sarcoidosis
    B. chlamydial infection
    C. histoplasmosis
    D. drugs
    E. all of the above

41. Increased pigmentation is usually associated with
    A. ultraviolet exposure in combination with contact with coal tar products
    B. percutaneous absorption of monobenzylether of hydroquinone (a rubber oxidant)
    C. freezing of cutaneous lesions with liquid nitrogen
    D. inhalation of various phenolic vapors (paratertiary butylphenol)
    E. none of the above

42. Scarring of the scalp with destruction of hair follicles leads to permanent baldness in which of the following?
    A. bismuth toxicity
    B. localized psoriasis of the scalp

C. excessive ionizing radiation
D. typhoid fever
E. hypothyroidism

43. Concerning pemphigus, which of the following statements is *incorrect*?

    A. pemphigus vulgaris and pemphigus vegetans are characterized by deep, suprabasal intraepidermal bullae
    B. pemphigus foliaceus and pemphigus erythematosus are characterized by superficial intraepidermal bullae
    C. deeper forms of pemphigus are less life-threatening than the superficial forms
    D. the exact etiology of pemphigus is unknown
    E. even in the corticosteroid era, the mortality rate of pemphigus vulgaris has remained high

44. Pemphigus vulgaris is characterized by

    A. a rounding up of epidermal cells resulting from a loss of adhesion between these cells (acantholysis)
    B. the lesions do not itch but can be very painful
    C. Nikolsky's sign (when firm pressure with the finger is exerted on normal skin, the epidermis slides off, owing to its generally poor attachment to the underlying dermis)
    D. the bullae typically arise from noninflammatory bases
    E. all of the above

45. Erythema multiforme is a cutaneous reaction pattern that may be provoked by

    A. viral infections
    B. bacterial infections
    C. drug ingestion
    D. endocrine factors
    E. all of the above

46. Which of the following corresponds with the description of erythema multiforme (bullosum)?

    A. eruption is characterized by the distinctive target, or iris, lesion
    B. multiple etiologic and triggering causes

C. the palms and soles are characteristically involved
D. the eruption is usually symptomless
E. all of the above

47. Which of the following statements concerning herpes gestationis is *incorrect*?

    A. the etiologic agent is related to the herpes group viruses
    B. morphologic similarity with cutaneous lesions is observed in bullous pemphigoid
    C. tendency towards remission following and between pregnancies
    D. significant fetal death and premature deliveries
    E. systemic corticosteroid therapy provides the only consistent benefit

48. A small proportion of patients given the antihypertensive drug hydralazine developed a drug-induced reaction very similar to

    A. toxic erythema
    B. systemic lupus erythematosus
    C. erythroderma
    D. erythema nodosum
    E. angioedema

49. Porphyria cutanea tarda as a result of exposure to hexachlorobenzene is characterized by which of the following?

    A. increased skin fragility
    B. blisters
    C. hypertrichosis
    D. hyperpigmentation
    E. all of the above

50. Granuloma pyogenicum is characterized by all of the following *except*

    A. bright red to reddish-brown vascular lesion
    B. most commonly found on the finger, hand, leg, or back
    C. often preceded by minor trauma
    D. the lesions bleed easily
    E. an infectious cause has been identified

Occupational Diseases of the Skin / 79

51. Keratoacanthoma is characterized by all of the following *except*
    A. the role of pitch and tar in the production of this lesion in industrial workers is well established
    B. it occurs more frequently on light-exposed areas
    C. the tumor occurs most frequently in persons under 20 years of age
    D. there is a higher incidence in smokers than in nonsmokers
    E. most tumors regress spontaneously

Directions: Each group of questions below consists of five lettered headings followed by a list of numbered words or phrases. For each numbered word or phrase select the one heading that is most closely related to it.

Questions 52 through 56

   A. Pustule
   B. Bulla
   C. Papule
   D. Wheal
   E. Macule

52. a transient, slightly raised, and usually flat lesion; urticaria
53. a flat, circumscribed area of altered skin color; neurofibromatosis
54. a small, circumscribed elevation of the skin; sarcoidosis
55. similar to a vesicle but larger (more than 5 mm in diameter); contact dermatitis
56. a collection of pus; vaccinia

Questions 57 through 61

   A. Nodule
   B. Vesicle
   C. Sclerosis
   D. Plaque
   E. Scar

57. a flat-topped palpable lesion; mycosis fungoides

58. a solid, circumscribed elevation whose greater part lies beneath the skin surface; lymphoma
59. a small (less than 5 mm in diameter), circumscribed, fluid-containing elevation; dermatitis herpetiformis
60. a circumscribed or diffuse hardening or induration of the skin; morphea
61. a permanent lesion that results from the process of repair by replacement with connective tissue; mutilations on the digits, leprosy

Questions 62 through 66

   A. Fissures
   B. Scale
   C. Crust
   D. Ulcer
   E. Excoriation

62. a shallow abrasion often caused by scratching; atopic eczema
63. linear cleavages in the skin that may be painful; perleche
64. a dried exudate; impetigo
65. thickened, loose, readily detached fragments of stratum corneum; psoriasis
66. an excavation due to loss of tissue, including the epidermal surface

Questions 67 through 71

   A. Albinism
   B. Vitiligo
   C. Freckles (ephelides)
   D. Addison's disease
   E. Mongolian spot

67. localized increase in melanogenesis; there is no increase in the number of melanocytes
68. an autosomal recessive disorder, characterized by a lack of pigment production by melanocytes in the epidermis, hair bulb, and eye
69. hormonally-mediated increase in melano-

genesis. Melanin deposition is increased mainly in the flexures and in the mucous membranes

70. an area of acquired cutaneous depigmentation due to loss of normal melanocyte function

71. localized increase in numbers of dermal melanocytes. A type of blue naevus frequently seen over the sacrum

Questions 72 through 76

A. Alopecia areata
B. Trichotillomania
C. Tinea capitis
D. Luetic alopecia
E. None of the above

72. "moth-eaten" scalp alopecia beginning in the occipital hair is characteristic

73. a compulsive desire to pull, twist, and tug at scalp hair; emotional factors are always present

74. scaly patches of different sizes in which broken hairs are seen; it occurs almost exclusively in children

75. loss of hair in round or oval well-defined patches, without inflammation; scaling or scarring; temporary arrest of growth or loss of nails

76. scalp scrapings and hairs should be examined microscopically and cultured to demonstrate the etiologic agent

Questions 77 through 81

A. Ichthyosis
B. Miliaria
C. Hidradenitis suppurativa
D. Herpetic whitlow
E. Hyperhidrosis

77. vesicular dermatitis secondary to trapping of sweat at some point in the skin

78. a tender, inflammatory, abscesslike swelling in the affected apocrine area

79. usually considered to be a feature of thyrotoxicosis

80. a disorder of keratinization characterized by excessive dry and scaling skin

81. the disease is common to the medical and dental professions; multiple discrete vesicles are seen

Questions 82 through 86

A. Antimalarials
B. Iodides and bromides
C. Penicillamine
D. β-Blockers
E. Coumarins

82. pemphiguslike eruption

83. psoriasiform eruption

84. alopecia

85. acneiform eruption

86. lichen planuslike eruption

Questions 87 through 91

A. Strawberry nevus
B. Cavernous hemangioma
C. Portwine stain
D. Acquired nevi
E. Dermal melanocytoma

87. a benign, spontaneously appearing neoplasm without hereditary influence; striking and characteristic color range, varying from blue-gray to royal blue; may be confused with malignant melanoma

88. vascular malformation present at, or appearing shortly after, birth; within the first three years of life most will begin to involute spontaneously

89. usually are not apparent at birth but first appear during infancy; may show progressive enlargement

90. lesions are usually present at birth; little tendency to involution; may be the cutaneous manifestation of syndromes in which the viscera as well as the skin are involved

91. these lesions, with occasional exceptions, are absent at birth; appear to be genetically determined; wide variations in form and color

Questions 92 through 96

   A. Seborrheic keratosis
   B. Pigmented actinic keratosis
   C. Bowen's tumor
   D. Kaposi's sarcoma
   E. Leukoplakia

92. scaly hyperpigmented lesions, sometimes ulcerated, which develop on exposed skin

93. a benign proliferation of epidermal cells; the very superficial "stuck onto" appearance is a helpful differential point

94. more common on areas of the skin protected from light; there is a possibility that all cases are due to arsenic

95. multiple dermal plaques, nodules, and tumors—more frequent on the lower extremities; prevalence of the disease has been noted in patients whose occupations required them to stand for long periods of time

96. characterized by patches on the lips and on any of the mucous membranes of the body; any form of chronic irritation may produce oral lesions

Questions 97 through 101

   A. Nystatin
   B. Griseofulvin
   C. Neomycin
   D. Methoxsalen
   E. Benzyl benzoate

97. ringworm of the scalp

98. oral candidiasis

99. scabicide

100. may be useful in vitiligo

101. topical antibacterial agent

Directions: Each set of lettered headings below is followed by a list of numbered words or phrases. For each numbered word or phrase select

   A. if the item is associated with A only
   B. if the item is associated with B only
   C. if the item is associated with both A and B
   D. if the item is associated with neither A nor B

Questions 102 through 106

   A. Rheumatoid arthritis
   B. Psoriatic arthritis
   C. Both
   D. Neither

102. associated cutaneous lesions

103. occasionally subcutaneous nodules

104. morning stiffness is a common complaint

105. dramatic response to colchicine

106. associated with urethritis

Questions 107 through 111

   A. Direct irritant contact dermatitis
   B. Allergic contact dermatitis
   C. Both
   D. Neither

107. generally affects only a few workers

108. prior exposure to substance is essential

109. the onset is rapid (4–12 hours) after contact

110. everyone is susceptible in varying degrees to appropriate concentrations

111. properly performed patch tests are reliable

Questions 112 through 116

   A. Erysipeloid
   B. Erysipelas
   C. Both
   D. Neither

112. commonly occurs on the hand or fingers of butchers, fishermen, and others handling raw fish, poultry, and meat products

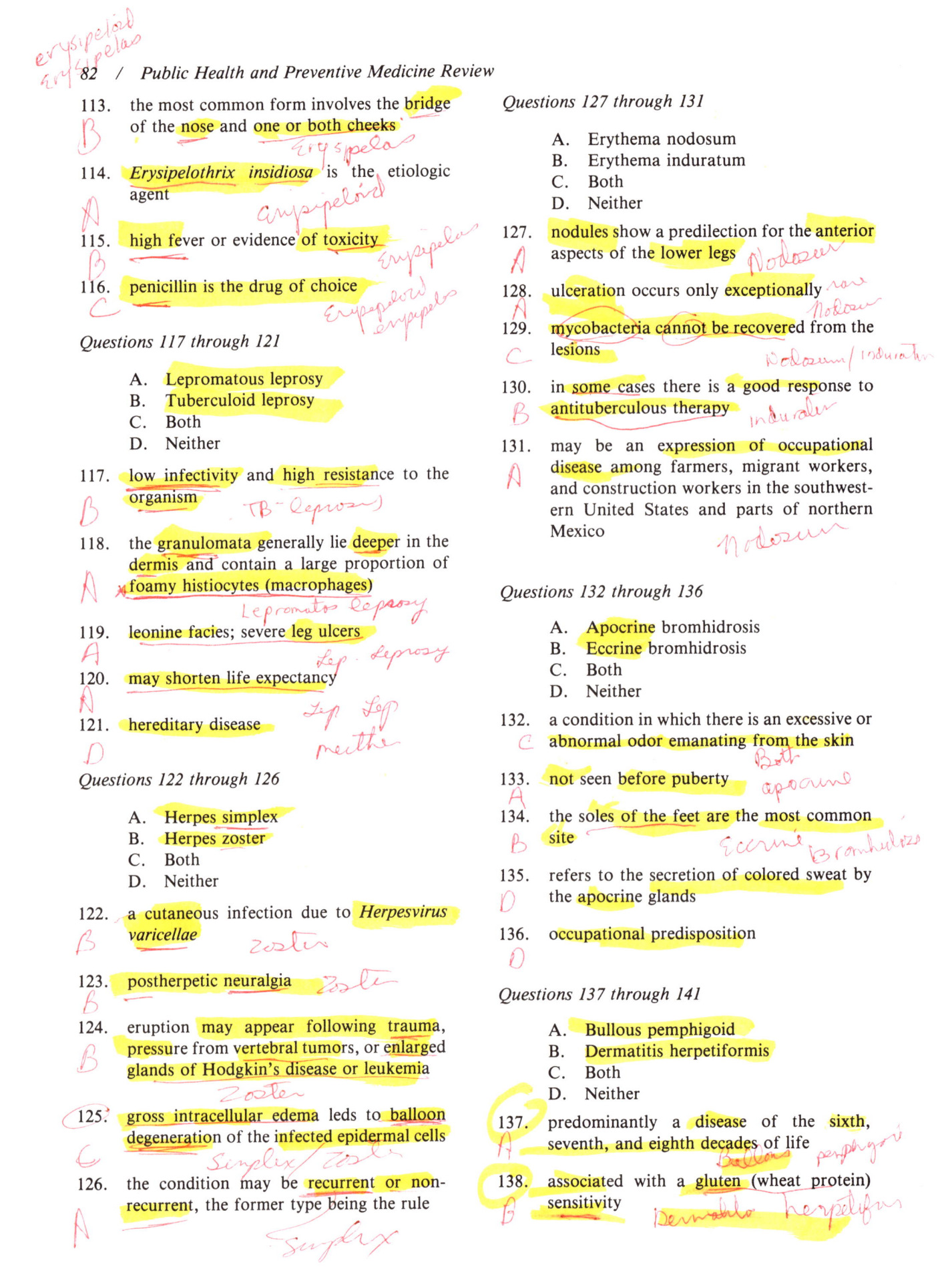

113. the most common form involves the bridge of the nose and one or both cheeks

114. *Erysipelothrix insidiosa* is the etiologic agent

115. high fever or evidence of toxicity

116. penicillin is the drug of choice

Questions 117 through 121

    A. Lepromatous leprosy
    B. Tuberculoid leprosy
    C. Both
    D. Neither

117. low infectivity and high resistance to the organism

118. the granulomata generally lie deeper in the dermis and contain a large proportion of foamy histiocytes (macrophages)

119. leonine facies; severe leg ulcers

120. may shorten life expectancy

121. hereditary disease

Questions 122 through 126

    A. Herpes simplex
    B. Herpes zoster
    C. Both
    D. Neither

122. a cutaneous infection due to *Herpesvirus varicellae*

123. postherpetic neuralgia

124. eruption may appear following trauma, pressure from vertebral tumors, or enlarged glands of Hodgkin's disease or leukemia

125. gross intracellular edema leds to balloon degeneration of the infected epidermal cells

126. the condition may be recurrent or non-recurrent, the former type being the rule

Questions 127 through 131

    A. Erythema nodosum
    B. Erythema induratum
    C. Both
    D. Neither

127. nodules show a predilection for the anterior aspects of the lower legs

128. ulceration occurs only exceptionally

129. mycobacteria cannot be recovered from the lesions

130. in some cases there is a good response to antituberculous therapy

131. may be an expression of occupational disease among farmers, migrant workers, and construction workers in the southwestern United States and parts of northern Mexico

Questions 132 through 136

    A. Apocrine bromhidrosis
    B. Eccrine bromhidrosis
    C. Both
    D. Neither

132. a condition in which there is an excessive or abnormal odor emanating from the skin

133. not seen before puberty

134. the soles of the feet are the most common site

135. refers to the secretion of colored sweat by the apocrine glands

136. occupational predisposition

Questions 137 through 141

    A. Bullous pemphigoid
    B. Dermatitis herpetiformis
    C. Both
    D. Neither

137. predominantly a disease of the sixth, seventh, and eighth decades of life

138. associated with a gluten (wheat protein) sensitivity

139. acantholysis (a rounding up of epidermal cells resulting from a loss of adhesion between these cells) is present

140. does not respond to systemic steroids

141. blistering disease

Questions 142 through 146

A. Basal cell carcinoma
B. Squamous cell carcinoma
C. Both
D. Neither

142. the commonest form of cutaneous malignancy

143. localized lymphadenitis may be present, and metastases should be sought

144. most common on light-exposed areas, particularly the vermillion of the lower lip

145. Gorlin's syndrome (a genetically determined condition)

146. spontaneously resolving tumor

Directions: For each of the incomplete statements below, ONE or MORE of the completions given is correct. In each case select

A. if only 1, 2, and 3 are correct
B. if only 1 and 3 are correct
C. if only 2 and 4 are correct
D. if only 4 is correct
E. if all are correct

147. The Koebner's (isomorphic) phenomenon (in which lesions will at times form precisely along a line of trauma) may be observed in

1. psoriasis
2. common wart (verruga vulgaris)
3. lichen planus
4. vitiligo

148. Vesicles are observed in

1. herpes zoster
2. rubella
3. dermatitis herpetiformis
4. measles

149. "Routine" preemployment patch-testing should be avoided because of

1. its high cost
2. the possibility of causing "specific hardening" of the skin
3. the frequency of secondary infections
4. medicolegal reasons

150. Which of the following compounds may cause occupational acne?

1. insoluble cutting oils
2. chlorinated hydrocarbons
3. coal tar derivatives
4. iodides

151. Which of the following statements about allergic eczematous contact dermatitis is (are) correct?

1. the acute stage is characterized by erythema, papules, vesicles, edema
2. thickening, scaling, and hyperpigmentation are characteristics of the chronic stage
3. when used correctly, patch tests are invaluable in identifying sensitizers causing allergic contact dermatitis
4. in industry, workers should be screened before given jobs in which dermatitis is a well-known risk

152. Which of the following statements about factitial dermatitis (dermatitis artefacta) is (are) correct?

1. there are inexplicable fluctuations in the severity of the lesions
2. bizarre configuration of the lesions is common
3. there is a temporary response to each new treatment
4. an emotional disturbance is the prominent issue

153. The positive diagnosis of leprosy is based on the

1. clinical appearance
2. demonstration of impairment of tactile sensitivity in a skin lesion
3. presence of *Mycobacterium leprae*
4. specific serologic test for leprosy

84 / Public Health and Preventive Medicine Review

154. Which of the following statements about the lepromin test (Mitsuda) is (are) correct?
    1. it is completely negative in the presence of lepromatous leprosy
    2. it is variably positive in tuberculoid leprosy
    3. it is sometimes positive in persons who have never been in contact with the leprosy bacillus
    4. a positive result indicates resistance to leprosy bacilli

155. Which of the following statements about leprosy therapy is (are) correct?
    1. most patients can, with perfect safety, be treated in their own homes
    2. Dapsone is the drug of choice for widespread use
    3. orthopedic and plastic procedures may be indicated
    4. the value of BCG vaccination as a prophylactic measure against leprosy is still in dispute

156. Hyperpigmentation may be observed in which of the following?
    1. pregnancy
    2. haemochromatosis
    3. Cushing's syndrome
    4. scleroderma

157. Anhidrosis without obvious skin disease can occur in association with
    1. multiple sclerosis
    2. hypothyroidism
    3. hypothalamic lesions
    4. heat stroke

158. Which of the following systemic reactions may be due to application of local glucocorticoids?
    1. posterior subcapsular cataracts
    2. peptic ulcer disease
    3. skin atrophy
    4. suppression of growth in children

159. Which of the following relating to sarcoidosis is (are) correct?
    1. subcutaneous infiltrations; tumorlike lesions
    2. micropapular eruption around the facial orifices
    3. the cause is unknown
    4. the Kveim test is used to confirm the diagnosis

160. Malignant tumors include
    1. squamous cell carcinoma
    2. basal cell carcinoma
    3. melanoma
    4. Bowen's disease

161. Association with an occult malignancy is not uncommon in
    1. dermatomyositis
    2. scleroderma
    3. acanthosis nigricans
    4. Reiter's syndrome

162. Which of the following statements about malignant melanoma is (are) correct?
    1. incidence is latitude-dependent
    2. long "disease-free" interval after removal of primary tumor and development of clinical metastasis
    3. high rate of spontaneous regression
    4. depigmentation at sites distant to the tumor and uveitis (inflammation of the melanocytes of the choroid of the eye) have been observed

163. Benign tumors include
    1. seborrheic keratosis
    2. pyogenic granuloma
    3. keratoacanthoma
    4. histiocytoma

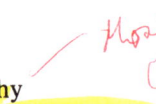

Answers and Explanations
Occupational Diseases of the Skin

1. **E.** A number of systemic disease states may be associated with persistent and severe pruritus of clinically normal skin. This may be a presenting feature of the systemic condition. Although psoriasis has been said to be asymptomatic, a proportion of patients with actively developing lesions complain of pruritus. (16:34)

2. **E.** Lack of cleanliness, either personal or environmental, is probably the most frequent cause of occupational dermatitis. (40:57)

3. **D.** In 1979, Department of Labor statistics indicated that almost one half of the nearly 150,000 cases of occupational diseases in the United States were skin conditions. This fraction has remained relatively constant for several years. The lost time for most cases is not great, but the total cost is considerable: recent estimates have suggested a figure of $30,000,000 annually, considering the cost of less efficient replacement workers, medical and indemnity costs, and insurance. (34:161)

4. **D.** Most occupational skin diseases are caused by irritating chemicals. These agents cause dermatitis by direct action on the normal skin at the site of contact, if they are permitted to act in sufficient intensity or quantity for a sufficient time. Any normal skin will thus react to a primary irritant if these conditions are met. (40:32)

5. **E.** Depending on the specific circumstances, there are a number of measures, including those listed, that can be instituted to help prevent occupational skin diseases. However, one must not only make rules but also see that they are complied with and are practical. (16:1013)

6. **E.** Occupational dermatoses exhibit considerable morphologic variety. Their appearance and pattern rarely indicate the provoking substance but may provide a clue as to a class of materials being encountered. Diagnosis depends upon appearance and location, but mostly upon history. Supervening infections or undesirable therapeutic effects make the diagnosis more difficult. With few exceptions, most of the morphologic patterns associated with occupational skin diseases can also result from non-occupational agents. (40:48)

7. **D.** Contact dermatitis is the most common pattern of occupational dermatoses. (40:35)

8. **A.** In 1978 the Standards Advisory Committee on cutaneous hazards identified high-risk industries on the basis of the incidence of skin diseases. The leading industry of this group was leather tanning and finishing, most likely the result of the large number of irritants and sensitizers used. Poultry dressing plants were second, due to the constant wetness of this work, which also is present in fresh or frozen packaged fish industries. Solvents and plastics materials are the chief culprits in adhesives and sealants and boat building and repairing. In landscape and horticulture, plants, especially those of the rhus group, are responsible for most of the cases. (1:829)

9. **A.** The disease is produced by the penetration of sharp needles of the sugar cane bark into the hair follicles of sugar cane workers, as described in Cuba by Pardo Castello. (15:228)

10. **E.** A study of allergic contact dermatitis revealed that nickel is one of the substances that produced the greatest number of clinically significant patch-test reactions. It has been considered that nickel produced more instances of contact dermatitis than did all the other metals put together. Nickel is found in coins, cutlery, cooking implements, gardening and motoring equipment, jewelry, and household furniture. There is evidence that ingesting trace amounts in the diet may play a part in perpetuating the skin lesions. (31:78)

11. **D.** Lichen planus is normally fairly easily diagnosed on clinical grounds, and histopathologic study will confirm the diagnosis in a typical case or enable a diagnosis to be made in difficult circumstances. (31:43)

12. **E.** Methotrexate therapy is probably the most successful treatment for this condition. Synthetic retinoids given systemically have produced encouraging results in some patients. Vitamin A therapy is reported to be effective in many cases. Ultraviolet-light treatment, as used for psoriasis, has not been helpful. (16:264)

13. **B.** An initial single plaque, called the "herald plaque," may appear anywhere on the body. This lesion commonly precedes the generalized eruption of pityriasis rosea by several days or weeks. (16:817)

14. **D.** Recurrences are unusual. A viral cause has been hypothesized because of the relatively short course of the disease, seasonal incidence, and outbreaks in institutions. There is no specific therapy. Spontaneous resolution usually occurs within a few weeks. (16:817)

15. **C.** Reiter's disease occurs most often in young adult males. The disease also occurs in females and children. Arthritis of the major weight-bearing joints, usually short-lived conjunctivitis, and nonspecific urethritis are symptoms. The cause of Reiter's syndrome has not been firmly established. There is no specific test. An increased erythrocyte sedimentation rate may be present. (16:1327)

16. **E.** Xanthomata is a metabolic disorder. The yellowish papules or nodules contain cholesterol. (31:229)

17. **C.** Psoriasis is commoner in northern climates and in the winter. Genetic factors play a role in the pathogenesis of psoriasis, and a high proportion of patients have a family history. The sexes are affected equally and the onset may be at any age. (52:58)

18. **D.** Characteristic pruritus is the cardinal feature of the disease. Most patients with atopic dermatitis have a positive family history of the atopic triad (dermatitis, asthma, and allergic rhinitis). The typical facial pallor seen in patients with atopic disease may reflect this associated paradoxical cutaneous vascular response. (31:68)

19. **D.** The etiology is unknown. Nummular eczema occurs at any age but particularly in tense middle-aged persons. It may also present as a manifestation of atopic dermatitis in children under the age of 10. (31:83)

20. **E.** Acne vulgaris is the most common of all skin conditions. (31:85)

21. **E.** Stasis dermatitis is characterized by an area of dermatitis on the lower legs, commonly seen in association with venous insufficiency or frank ulceration. The use of topical steroids is not recommended. (31:84)

22. **E.** A furuncle is an acute painful infection of a hair follicle caused by *Staphylococcus aureus*. A variety of systemic host factors is associated with furunculosis. These include obesity and blood dyscrasias. Whether diabetes mellitus predisposes to furunculosis is still controversial. (52:107)

23. **E.** Lupus miliaris disseminatus faciei is a papular eruption of the face, running a chronic course and terminating with spontaneous involution. There is no evidence supporting a linking to tuberculosis. (16:1487)

24. **B.** The cause of dermatitis herpetiformis is not known. (52:156)

25. **E.** Anogenital warts must be differentiated from the moist, flat papules of secondary syphilis—condyloma lata. The peak incidence of warts occurs during the second decade of life; possibly 10% of teenagers have warts. Trauma plays some factor in inoculation, because warts often occur at pressure points and in scratches. (16:1631)

26. **D.** The diagnosis is easily made by the distinctive clinical appearance of the lesions, by stained smears of the expressed core, and by biopsy (rarely required). This disorder is not uncommon in beauty specialists and masseurs who contract it from their clients, and also transmit it to them. The fully developed lesion is an umbilicated papule, and most patients have multiple lesions. The development of new lesions by autoinoculation is common. The mode of person-to-person spread is unknown. Most cases resolve spontaneously in six to nine months, but some may persist for three years or longer. (52:157)

27. **E.** Erythrasma, caused by *Corynebacterium minitissimum*, is characterized by reddish-brown areas of skin, commonly in body flexures, particularly in the groin. It does not appear to be contagious and, if untreated, it spreads slowly with a well-demarcated advancing edge. It is asymptomatic. The etiologic agent of thrush: *Candida albicans*; of kerion: *Tricophyton verrucosum;* of ringworm: *Tricophyton rubrum*. (31:109)

28. **E.** In those whose hands are habitually immersed in water, candida paronchia is an occupational hazard. The incidence of candida vaginitis, with extension to the vulva, increases in pregnancy.

Intraoral thrush is seen as a whitish loose membrane on the inner surface of the cheeks, or on the palate of babies, children, or young adults. Superficial glossitis may appear in adults as a beefy-red, smooth tongue. (16:1518)

29. E. The following occupations predispose to candida infection: homemaking, bartending, and baking. (52:142)

30. E. Griseofulvin tablets are given, 1 g daily for two to three weeks, but if lesions number only one or two, Whitfield's ointment or clotrimaxole (Canesten) 1% cream can be used instead. (52:138)

31. B. This is a chronic, symptomless fungus infection. The causative organism is known as *Pityrosporum orbiculare* in its yeastlike form, and as *Malassezia furfur* when it becomes hyphal. (52:142)

32. E. Skin scrapings for direct microscopy and examination under Wood's light for pale yellow fluorescence can both be used to identify the organism. (52:142)

33. B. The main complaint is itching, worse at night; if this symptom is not pathognomonic it is highly suggestive of scabies. Diagnosis is made by recognizing the multiform character of the lesions and their locale. The characteristic lesion is the burrow. (16:1659)

34. D. Endemic typhus is transmitted to humans by the rat flea. (16:1662)

35. E. Although the title emphasizes involvement of the beard, other hairy areas such as the thighs may also become affected. On the face, the condition is usually secondary to a nasal infection. (52:108)

36. E. Among the predisposing factors are infected nostrils or ears, dirty fingernails or towels, or infection from an existing condition such as pediculosis capitis, scabies, or eczematous conditions. Diabetes is not a predisposing cause. (52:106)

37. A. Skin lesions are present in only 50% of cases. Other clinical signs are legion, as any organ may be affected. The effect of sunlight on a skin lesion may result in the development of an acute exacerbation. Drug reactions to sulphonamides and penicillin, among others, may also produce the same effect. Women are more often affected than men, in a ratio of 8:1. Treatment is usually based on systemic corticosteroids together with, in some cases, an immunosuppressive agent. (52:199)

38. E. Antibiotics must be avoided, as they may disseminate the disease. Unlike systemic lupus erythematosus, lesions in the scalp can destroy the hair bulbs, leaving a permanent scarring alopecia. The presence of red, scaly discs on light-exposed skin is strongly suggestive, and if a scale is removed from a lesion its under-surface will show the pathognomonic plugs that have occupied the pilosebaceous follicles. (52:195)

39. A. Chelation therapy with intravenous EDTA in patients with calcinosis universalis has not produced clinical benefit. Corticosteroids play the major role in the therapy of dermatomyositis. (16:1303)

40. E. It is symptomatic of a bacterial, viral, or fungal disease; a drug reaction; or a concomitant condition. Streptococcal conditions are probably the commonest cause. Acute erythema nodosum associated with bilateral hilar lymphadenopathy and negative tuberculin test is now generally accepted as an expression of sarcoidosis. Erythema nodosum may be associated with deep fungous infections such as histoplasmosis. Bedsonia may play a role in erythema nodosum. (31:152)

41. A. A number of substances and conditions may alter pigment formation. The changes that occur—darkening or lightening—are based on interference of the biochemical synthesis of melanin. Increased pigmentation is usually associated with ultraviolet exposure alone, or such exposure in combination with contact with coal tar products. Pigment loss (leukoderma) may result from, among other causes, absorption of a rubber oxidant (hydroquinone). (40:36)

42. C. Excessive ionizing radiation causes scarring of the scalp with destruction of hair follicles, which leads to permanent baldness. Bismuth toxicity may produce alopecia which is reversible on treatment with chelating agents. Localized psoriasis of the scalp may cause alopecia, but a return to normal hair pattern is the rule. Complete regrowth is the rule in cases of postfebrile hair loss. Frank hypothyroidism always causes some hair loss of the scalp, eyebrows, and secondary sexual hair. Thyroid replacement therapy usually results in complete resolution of hair loss. (16:396)

43. C. The superficial forms of pemphigus are the less life-threatening. Pemphigus vulgaris was considered universally fatal before the development of corticosteroid therapy. (16:310)

44. E. Pemphigus vulgaris frequently begins insidiously, with the slow development of raw areas and shallow erosions of the mucous membranes. Involvement of the skin tends to come later. The patient may therefore complain first of mouth ulcers or genital discomfort. (31:192)

45. **E.** In many cases, no etiologic or precipitating factor can be identified. (31:200)

46. **E.** The characteristic target (iris) lesion, which consists of a clear red area as a periphery surrounding a pale zone and a central livid area that may contain a bulla or a vesicle. Although patients occasionally complain of burning or itching, the eruption is usually symptomless. (16:295)

47. **A.** The etiology of herpes gestationis is unknown. It is not related to the herpes viruses group. Papulovesicular lesions are characteristic. Infants born of affected mothers receiving high doses of prednisone should be carefully examined by a neonatologist for evidence of adrenal insufficiency. (16:325)

48. **B.** Some of the commoner drugs known to induce a reaction similar to systemic lupus erythematosus are: hydralazine, methyldopa, griseofulvin, oral contraceptives, penicillin, phenylbutazone, procaine amide, sulphonamides, and diphenylhydantoin. (31:216)

49. **E.** Biochemical studies confirmed that individuals with these manifestations had developed porphyria cutanea tarda as a result of exposure to hexachlorobenzene. (37:564)

50. **E.** An infectious cause is implied by its name, but proof of this is lacking. The lesion often develops after trauma, commonly on the fingers. (16:728)

51. **C.** The tumor occurs most frequently between the ages of 60 and 65. Sunlight is thought to be a factor in the production of some keratoacanthomas. Although most tumors regress spontaneously, treatment should be by excision biopsy to provide the entire lesion for histologic study. (31:279)

52. **D.** Wheal: a rounded or flat-topped elevation in the skin that is characteristically evanescent, disappearing within hours. (16:21)

53. **E.** Macule: a circumscribed area of change in normal skin color without elevation or depression of the surface relative to the surrounding skin. (16:20)

54. **C.** Papule: a solid, elevated lesion. Generally considered to be less than 1 cm in diameter, and most of the lesion is above the plane of the surrounding skin rather than deep within it. (16:20)

55. **B.** Bulla: a circumscribed, elevated lesion that contains fluid, with a diameter greater than 0.5 cm. (16:21)

56. **A.** Pustule: a circumscribed elevation of the skin that contains a purulent exudate. (16:22)

57. **D.** Plaque: an elevation above the skin surface that occupies a relatively large surface area in comparison with its height above the skin. Frequently formed by confluence of papules. (16:16)

58. **A.** Nodule: a palpable, solid, round, or ellipsoidal lesion deeper than a papule. Can be located in the dermis or subcutaneous tissue. (16:16)

59. **B.** Vesicle (blister): a circumscribed, elevated lesion that contains fluid. (16:17)

60. **C.** Sclerosis: a circumscribed or diffuse hardening or induration of the skin. (16:18)

61. **E.** Scar: occurs wherever ulceration has taken place and reflects the pattern of healing in these areas. (16:18)

62. **E.** Excoriation: superficial excavation of epidermis that may be linear or punctate and result from scratching. (31:6)

63. **A.** Fissures: frequently noted at the angles of the mouth. (16:18)

64. **C.** Crust: results when serum, blood, or purulent exudate dries on the skin surface. (31:6)

65. **B.** Scales: a component of a variety of conditions (psoriasis, tinea, pityriasis rosea, secondary or tertiary syphilis). (31:6)

66. **D.** Ulcers: lesions in which there has been destruction of the epidermis and the upper (papillary) dermis. (31:6)

67. **C.** In freckles, groups of melanocytes produce an abnormally large amount of melanin in response to sunlight. There is no increase in the number of melanocytes. (52:167)

68. **A.** In albinism, the melanocyte either lacks the enzymes necessary for melanin pigment synthesis, or these are present in an abnormal nonfunctional form. (52:163)

69. **D.** In Addison's disease, melanin deposition is increased, mainly in the flexures and in the mucous membranes. (52:167)

70. **B.** In vitiligo, there is a localized loss of melanocytes. (52:164)

71. **E.** The mongolian spot is also a type of blue nevus. (52:170)

72. **D.** Some patients with secondary syphilis present with a diffuse "moth-eaten" pattern of hair loss, but its relationship to the other signs and symp-

toms at this stage is unclear. Hair regrowth follows adequate antibiotic therapy. (59:57)

73. **B.** Trichotillomania is characterized by an uncontrollable desire to pull out one's own hair. Mild or severe frustrations and anxieties may exist or, more rarely, a true psychosis may be present. (31:177)

74. **C.** The onset of tinea capitis varies according to the fungus involved. Generally, however, it is gradual. (52:140)

75. **A.** Alopecia areata often occurs in several members of a family. There are also reports of cases in identical twins. (52:224)

76. **C.** All suspected cases of tinea capitis and contacts should be examined under Wood's light. However, only lesions due to *Microsporum canis* or *Microsporum audovini* will show bright blue-green fluorescence. (31:180)

77. **B.** Miliaria involves vesicular lesions resulting from occlusion of sweat glands. Common in hot, humid environments. (16:477)

78. **C.** Hidradenitis suppurativa is a functional and structural abnormality of apocrine sweat glands. Deep-seated inflammatory lesions are located chiefly in the axillae and groins. (16:480)

79. Hyperhidrosis is an overproduction of sweat that can be due to heat or emotional stimuli or to endocrinologic or neurologic disorders. (16:464)

80. **A.** In some types of ichthyosis the sweat glands are hypoplastic or absent, with resultant decreased sweating. (16:469)

81. **D.** Herpetic whitlow: Acute paronychia due to herpes simplex is an occupational hazard to doctors and nurses. (16:1594)

82. **C.** Penicillamine is used as a chelating agent and as an antirheumatic, and in a proportion of patients it causes a blistering eruption that is clinically, histologically, and immunologically identical to pemphigus vulgaris. (31:212)

83. **D.** B-blocker drugs, particularly practolol, can give rise to the "oculomucocutaneous syndrome," characterized by keratoconjunctivitis, a psoriasiform eruption, and many serious problems such as sclerosing peritonitis and pericarditis. (31:211)

84. **E.** Coumarins occasionally cause hair loss. (31:173)

85. **B.** Bromides and iodides may cause an acneiform eruption, but without the blackheads that occur in true acne. (52:93)

86. **A.** Complications of antimalarial therapy include lichen planuslike eruptions, yellow discoloration of the skin, retinopathy, pigmentation of the nails and palate, and depigmentation of the hair. (52:208)

87. **E.** Dermal melanocytoma (blue nevus) exhibits a specific histologic picture. (16:647)

88. **A.** Spontaneous involution of strawberry nevi usually occurs by the age of two or three years. (16:727)

89. **B.** Cavernous hemangiomas are characterized by tumorlike aggregates of dilated vessels or sinusoidal blood spaces in a delicate fibrous stroma. (16:730)

90. **C.** Nevus flammeus (port-wine stain). When located in the distribution of the trigeminal nerve there may be associated vascular anomalies in the eye, and leptomeninges and superficial calcifications in the brain. (16:732)

91. **D.** Acquired nevi (moles) are lesions that appear after birth and are proliferative aggregates of apparently normal melanocytes that appear to be hereditarily determined. (16:643)

92. **B.** Ultraviolet light can induce premalignant changes in the epidermis that are recognizable both clinically and histologically and are termed actinic keratoses, or senile keratoses. (31:261)

93. **A.** Seborrheic keratosis (basal cell papillamata) become commoner with increasing age. (31:276)

94. **C.** Bowen's carcinoma in situ: In the past, a high proportion of patients have had a history of arsenic ingestion, formerly an ingredient of "tonics" and "appetite stimulants." (31:263)

95. **D.** Kaposi's sarcoma is a neoplasm of multifocal origin that manifests primarily as multiple vascular nodules in the skin and other organs. (16:743)

96. **E.** Fair-skinned people are more likely to suffer leukoplakia. Male sufferers outnumber females. (52:217)

97. **B.** Griseofulvin is effective in the treatment of fungal infections of the skin, nails, and hair. It has no apparent effect on systemic fungal infections. (35:631)

98. **A.** Nystatin is used in the local treatment of moniliasis. Parenteral preparations are too irritating to be practicable in the treatment of systemic mycoses. (35:631)

99. **E.** Benzyl benzoate is effective in scabies. (35:633)

100. **D.** Psoralen induces hypersensitivity to ultraviolet light. The subsequent stimulation of melanin pigments may be useful in vitiligo. (35:633)

101. **C.** Neomycin (0.5% ointment) may be useful whem mixed gram-negative bacteria require local treatment. (35:631)

102. **B.** Psoriatic arthritis is associated with typical psoriatic lesions of the skin. (16:251)

103. **A.** Subcutaneous nodules near extensor surfaces, if found, strongly suggest rheumatoid arthritis. (16:251)

104. **C.** Morning stiffness is a common complaint in both conditions. (16:251)

105. **D.** Neither of these conditions will improve after treatment with colchicine. (16:251)

106. **D.** Urethritis is not associated with rheumatoid arthritis or with psoriatic arthritis. (16:251)

107. **B.** A sensitizer generally affects only a few workers. An irritant usually affects many workers. (31:75)

108. **B.** Allergic contact dermatitis occurs only in patients whose skin has previously been sensitized by contact with an allergen. (31:75)

109. **A.** A rapid onset (4–12 hours) after direct contact is characteristic of direct irritant contact dermatitis. In allergic contact dermatitis, onset is generally 24 hours or longer after exposure. (31:75)

110. **A.** In allergic contact dermatitis, only some persons are susceptible. (31:75)

111. **B.** Patch tests, if properly performed, are a reliable and useful method of testing for allergic contact hypersensitivity. (16:517)

112. **A.** Occurrence of the disease is limited almost exclusively to persons handling contaminated products. (16:1462)

113. **B.** The face is a common site of erysipela. A "butterfly" distribution is common. (16:1430)

114. **A.** *Erysipelothrix insidiosa*, a gram-positive rod, is the etiologic agent of erysipeloid. Erysipelas are due to group A, B, C, or G streptococci or *Staphylococcus aureus*. (16:1462)

115. **B.** Erysipeloid is not associated with high fever or evidences of toxicity. (16:1431)

116. **C.** Penicillin G is the drug of choice in the treatment of group A streptococcal skin infections. Penicillin in doses of 2 to 3 million units daily, for seven to 10 days, is the treatment for erysipeloid. (16:1437)

117. **B.** The tuberculoid form is associated with low infectivity and a high degree of natural resistance to the organism. The lepromatous type is associated with large numbers of easily identified microorganisms, a high degree of infectivity, and little natural resistance to the mycobacteria. (31:96)

118. **A.** In lepromatous leprosy the granulomata generally lie deeper in the dermis and contain a large proportion of macrophages. *Mycobacterium leprae* are present in large numbers in these cells. (31:97)

119. **A.** As the untreated lepromatous leprosy advances, among the features that develop are the following: thinning or loss of eyebrows and eyelashes and thickening of the ear lobes and of the skin of the face, with deepening of the lines of the forehead (leonine facies). Severe and intractable leg ulcers may develop. (52:124)

120. **A.** Lepromatous leprosy is the only type of leprosy that may shorten life expectancy. Death is more often due to renal damage in the form of chronic glomerulonephritis, chronic interstitial nephritis, or renal amyloidosis. (52:1494)

121. **D.** While congenital infections have been recorded, they are exceedingly rare and, for all intents and purposes, leprosy is not a hereditary disease in the true sense of the word. (15:1494)

122. **B.** Herpes zoster is caused by *Herpesvirus varicellae*. Herpes simplex is caused by *Herpesvirus hominis*. (31:107)

123. **B.** Postherpetic neuralgia occurs especially in old people and may be so distressing and chronic as to induce suicidal depression. It may, however, clear spontaneously in a few months. (52:152)

124. **B.** The eruption may appear following trauma, pressure from vertebral tumors, enlarged glands of Hodgkin's disease or leukemia, or infections such as meningitis. (52:151)

125. **C.** As in herpes simplex, the striking histologic feature of herpes zoster is balloon degeneration (the presence of grossly swollen, distorted cells in the epidermis). (31:107)

126. **A.** Herpes simplex is characterized by grouped vesicles on a red base, usually affecting the lips, face, or genitalia. The condition may be recurrent or nonrecurrent. (52:154)

127. **A.** Erythema nodosum is a syndrome of inflammatory cutaneous nodules usually limited to the extensor aspects of the limbs, particularly the lower legs. The sites of predilection of the erythema induratum lesions are the calves. (16:784, 1486)

128. **A.** Ulceration occurs only exceptionally in erythema nodosum. Recurring nodules and ulcers are observed in erythema induratum. (16:1486)

129. **C.** Mycobacteria cannot be recovered from erythema nodosum or erythema induratum. (16:1486)

130. **B.** In some cases there is a good response to antituberculous therapy in erythema induratum. However, this does not necessarily prove a tuberculosis etiology. (16:1486)

131. **A.** Erythema nodosum. (16:1550)

132. **C.** Bromhidrosis, or osmidrosis, is a condition in which there is an excessive or abnormal odor emanating from the skin. (16:473)

133. **A.** Apocrine bromhidrosis is not seen before puberty, since apocrine glands are functionless in the prepubertal period. (16:473)

134. **B.** Eccrine cromhidrosis results from bacterial action on keratin softened by sweating. The soles of the feet are the most common sites. (16:474)

135. **D.** Apocrine bromhidrosis refers to the secretion of colored sweat by the apocrine glands. (16:475)

136. **D.** There is no occupational or geographic predisposition. The problem may be more intense in the summer months because of increased eccrine sweating, which augments the production of axillary odor. (16:473)

137. **A.** Bullous pemphigoid occurs in elderly people. Dermatitis herpetiformis may start at any age, including childhood, but the second, third, or fourth decades are most common. (52:170)

138. **B.** Most patients (dermatitis herpetiformis) have an associated gluten-sensitive enteropathy, which is usually asymptomatic. (52:170)

139. **D.** Acantholysis is a histopathologic hallmark of the pemphigus group. It is absent in bullous pemphigoid and dermatitis herpetiformis. (52:170)

140. **B.** Dermatitis herpetiformis does not respond to steroids. Dapsone, diasone, and sulfonamides provide prompt improvement in the symptomatology of this condition. (52:170)

141. **C.** The outstanding clinical feature of bullous pemphigoid is the large, tense bullae. Blisters may attain considerable size. The primary lesion of dermatitis herpetiformis most commonly is a vesicle. (52:170)

142. **A.** Basal cell carcinomas (rodent ulcers, or basal cell epitheliomas) are the commonest form of skin cancer, accounting for approximately 70% of the total. (52:242)

143. **B.** Metastatic spread to the local draining lymph nodes and beyond will occur if the squamous cell carcinoma is not treated promptly. Basal cell carcinomas do not metastasize but they may cause extensive and distressing local destruction of soft tissue, cartilage, and even bone. (31:264)

144. **B.** A high proportion of squamous cell carcinomas arise on sun-damaged skin, particularly the vermillion of the lower lip. Basal cell carcinomas are seen predominantly on exposed sites commonly around the nose and the inner canthus. (31:264)

145. **A.** Gorlin's syndrome is characterized by the appearance of multiple basal cell carcinomas, jaw cysts, palmoplantar cutaneous pits, and skeletal abnormalities. (31:271)

146. **D.** Basal cell carcinomas and squamous cell carcinomas require treatment (surgical or radiotherapy). (31:246)

147. **E.** It is possible to partly explain the Koebner or isomorphic phenomenon in immunological terms. This phenomenon may also be seen occasionally in eczema. (31:33)

148. **B.** Vesicles are observed in herpes zoster (shingles) and dermatitis herpetiformis. Rubella and measles are characterized by a macular rash. (52:161)

149. **D.** Routine use of preemployment patch-testing as a screening procedure should be discouraged. The use of irritant concentrations in patch testing may sensitize an individual where no sensitivity existed previously. "Hardening" is a phenomenon in which a person allergic to a particular chemical becomes less reactive to it with constant exposure. (1:833)

150. **A.** Cutting oils are the most common cause of occupational acne. Tar acne is often accompanied by hyperpigmentation. The disease induced

by chlorinated hydrocarbons is characterized by its severity. (16:451)

151. **E.** The actual cause may be either a "primary irritant" or a "sensitizer." A primary irritant is a substance that will produce inflammation on first contact with the skin. (52:47)

152. **E.** Factitial dermatitis is characterized by bizarre lesions on any body site, deliberately initiated or aggravated by the patient. The patients primarily hurt themselves in order to deceive the physician and, in a way, to victimize her or him, although they may be unaware of that motivation. (16:1355)

153. **A.** The positive diagnosis of leprosy is based on the clinical appearance, together with either the demonstration of impairment of tactile sensitivity in a skin lesion or the presence of *Mycobacterium leprae*. There are no specific serologic tests for leprosy. (16:1503)

154. **E.** The lepromin test is used widely in leprosy. Reactions to lepromin are of two kinds: the early (Fernandez) reaction, which becomes positive in 48 hours, and the late (Mitsuda) reaction, read at four to five weeks. (35:305)

155. **E.** About 90% of patients are treated in their own homes. Dapsone is effective in all varieties of leprosy and relatively free from severe side effects. Physiotherapy and vocational training are part of the modern treatment of leprosy. Since BCG vaccination is of value in protecting children from tuberculosis, it may have a slight nonspecific effect in enhancing potential cell-mediated immunity against leprosy challenge. (16:1503)

156. **E.** Brownish patches may appear on the face of the pregnant woman (chloasma, melasma) that are due to the melanocyte-stimulating hormone of the pituitary gland. They disappear at the end of pregnancy. Occasionally, they appear in non-pregnant women. (52:179)

157. **E.** Anhidrosis without obvious skin disease can occur in association with hypothyroidism, dehydration, and heat stroke. It also occurs in association with disorders of the nervous system such as hypothalamic lesions, multiple sclerosis, and syringomyelia. (16:32)

158. **E.** The importance of adverse effects of topical corticosteroids are widely recognized. Skin atrophy is the most common adverse effect. (16:1757)

159. **E.** A papular eruption distributed around the facial orifices is characteristic. Deeper forms include nodules. The etiology is unknown. An intradermal test (Kveim-Siltbach) is available and is read at one month. When positive, a palpable nodule biopsy reveals sarcoid tissue. (31:228)

160. **E.** Squamous cell carcinoma is a malignant tumor derived from keratinocytes; despite the term "basal cell carcinoma," the cell type from which this tumor is derived has yet to be established. Melanoma is a malignant tumor of epidermal melanocytes. Bowen's tumor is a form of intraepidermal carcinoma in situ. (31:259)

161. **B.** Dermatomyositis may precede the development of the malignancy by months or even years. Acanthosis nigricans' commonest association is with gastrointestinal malignancies. (31:237)

162. **E.** There appears to be a fairly well-established relationship to latitude. Close to the equator, the melanoma incidence and mortality rate are higher. The tumor may remain at its local site in a nonmetastatic form for years prior to deep invasion and metastases. (16:641)

163. **E.** Seborrheic keratosis is a benign proliferation of epidermal cells. Pyogenic granuloma is a rapidly growing, benign tumor arising from the cutaneous vasculature. Keratoacanthoma is a rapidly growing and spontaneously resolving epidermal tumor. Histiocytoma is a quite benign lesion. (31:276)

CHAPTER SIX

Occupational Lung Disorders

Directions: Each of the questions or incomplete statements below is followed by five suggested answers or completions. Select the BEST answer in each case.

1. Which of the following is *not* a pneumoconiosis?

    A. siderosis
    B. argyrosiderosis
    C. silicosis
    D. sarcoidosis
    E. Shaver's disease

2. All of the following may cause pneumoconiosis *except*

    A. talc-associated minerals
    B. bauxite
    C. barium
    D. diatomaceous earth
    E. gypsum

3. Which of the following is composed of solid particles formed by combustion and condensation or chemical combination of substances in gaseous form?

    A. fumes
    B. dust
    C. mists
    D. gases
    E. vapors

4. Which of the following types of pneumoconiosis predisposes significantly to the development of tuberculosis?

    A. asbestos
    B. berylliosis
    C. aluminosis
    D. silicosis
    E. baritosis

5. Which of the following exhibits some, but not all, of the characteristics of "idiopathic" sarcoidosis and affects chiefly the lungs, although granulomas of the skin may occur in the absence of disease of the lungs and other organs?

    A. fibrocavernous tuberculosis
    B. miliary tuberculosis
    C. chronic beryllium disease
    D. bronchiectasis
    E. allergic bronchopulmonary aspergillosis

6. Shaver's disease is a fibrosis related to

    A. lead fume
    B. bauxite fume
    C. barite (compound of barium)
    D. soapstone (impure talcose rock)
    E. zircon

7. The finding of asbestos bodies in the sputum or lung biopsy is indicative of

    A. asbestosis
    B. pleural plaques

94 / Public Health and Preventive Medicine Review

C. malignant mesothelioma of pleura and peritoneum
D. exposure to asbestos
E. none of the above

8. Gradual onset of symptoms within hours of returning to work on Monday, tightness in the chest, dyspnea, cough, and emphysema point to

   A. bagassosis
   B. siderosis
   C. berylliosis
   D. silicosis
   E. byssinosis

9. The majority of patients suffering acute bagassosis will recover four to 12 weeks after

   A. oxygen administration
   B. streptomycin therapy
   C. antihistamine therapy
   D. being removed from exposure
   E. none of the above

Directions: Each group of questions below consists of five lettered headings followed by a list of numbered words or phrases. For each numbered word or phrase select the one heading that is most closely related to it.

Questions 10 through 14

   A. Stannosis
   B. Silo-fillers' disease
   C. Byssinosis
   D. Farmers' lung disease
   E. Siderosis

Inhalation of

10. the dusts of cotton

11. nitrogen oxide gases

12. dusts of moldy hay

13. iron oxide dust

14. tin oxide fumes

Directions: Each set of lettered headings below is followed by a list of numbered words or phrases. For each numbered word or phrase select

   A. if the item is associated with A only
   B. if the item is associated with B only
   C. if the item is associated with both A and B
   D. if the item is associated with neither A nor B

Questions 15 through 19

   A. "Idiopathic" sarcoidosis
   B. Beryllium disease
   C. Both
   D. Neither

15. history of occupational exposure

16. hypercalcemia

17. cystic changes in the bones of the hands and feet

18. involvement of the lachrymal and salivary glands

19. lymph node involvement

Directions: For each of the incomplete statements below, ONE or MORE of the completions given is correct. In each case select

   A. if only 1, 2, and 3 are correct
   B. if only 1 and 3 are correct
   C. if only 2 and 4 are correct
   D. if only 4 is correct
   E. if all are correct

Questions 20 through 25

20. Clinical features said to accompany lung disease of asbestos origin include

    1. shortness of breath
    2. dry rales
    3. pleuritic pain
    4. clubbing of fingers

21. Which of the following dusts can cause radiologic changes in the absence of disease?

    1. antimony
    2. barium
    3. iron
    4. tin

22. Clubbing of the fingers is associated with
    1. silicosis
    2. chromite pneumoconiosis
    3. talc pneumoconiosis
    4. calcium pneumoconiosis

23. The Kveim test would be positive in which of the following?
    1. papulonecrotic tuberculid
    2. chronic beryllium disease
    3. talc pneumoconiosis
    4. "idiopathic" sarcoidosis

24. There is no specific drug therapy for
    1. asbestosis
    2. diatomaceous earth pneumoconiosis
    3. silicosis
    4. woolsorters' disease

25. Skin tests are not of practical value in the diagnosis of
    1. farmers' lung disease
    2. histoplasmosis
    3. bagassosis
    4. coccidioidomycosis

Answers and Explanations
Occupational Lung Disorders

1. **D.** Sarcoidosis is widely regarded as a disorder of the immune system. Siderosis is caused by iron oxide dusts. The inhalation of iron oxide and silver produces the condition known as argyrosiderosis. Free silica causes a characteristic nodular, hyaline fibrosis. Shaver's disease is probably caused by a combined action of silica (quartz) and aluminum dust. (7:150)

2. **E.** Gypsum has been used for thousands of years as a building material. Gypsum does not cause a pneumoconiosis. "Talc" pneumoconiosis appears to consist of three different basic lesions: irregular quasinodular fibrosis, diffuse interstitial fibrosis, and foreign-body granulomas—depending upon the dominant composition of dust inhaled. Shaver's disease is bauxite pneumoconiosis. Barium is the cause of barium lung (baritosis). Diatomite is an amorphous form of silicon dioxide; the related disorder is called diatomite pneumoconiosis. (41:130)

3. **A.** Solid particles are generated by condensation from the gaseous state, generally after volatilization from molten materials. (45:3)

4. **D.** Silicosis is the only pneumoconiosis that predisposes to the development of tuberculosis. Although the incidence of tuberculosis in silicosis has fallen dramatically since the 1950s, it is still the most common complication. (21:343)

5. **C.** Tuberculosis is ruled out by appropriate study of sputum or gastric washings. Chronic beryllium disease, in contrast to Boeck's sarcoid, has not to date attacked the eye or tonsils. Skin lesions in the two diseases are identical in appearance. (21:32)

6. **B.** Fibrosis related to bauxite (aluminum oxide) fume is often known as Shaver's disease, after Shaver, who, with Ridell, described the association in 1947. Soapstone is a term loosely applied to impure talcose rocks containing variable amounts of talc and other minerals. (21:10)

7. **D.** The presence of asbestos bodies in sputum can be taken as evidence of exposure to asbestos but it does not imply disease. (61:101)

8. **E.** Characteristically, symptoms are first noticed on Monday mornings, when the cotton worker returns from a weekend away from exposure. (14:24)

9. **D.** The majority of patients suffering from acute bagassosis will recover four to 12 weeks after being removed from exposure. (41:380)

10. **C.** Although cotton dust is the most common cause of byssinosis, the disease is also caused by flax and hemp dusts. (19:217)

11. **B.** Silo-fillers' disease is the result of inhalation of nitrogen dioxide. (19:68)

12. **D.** The respiratory disease known as farmers' lung disease has been associated with inhalation of moldy hay, oats, barley, and millet grain. (21:375)

13. **E.** Siderosis is caused by the inhalation of iron oxide dust. (21:339)

14. **A.** Stannosis is caused by the inhalation of tin dusts or fumes. (21:340)

15. **B.** Beryllium disease is diagnosed on the basis of a history of occupational exposure to beryllium. (45:358)

16. **A.** Hypercalcemia is found in sarcoidosis. (45:124)

17. **A.** Cystic changes in the bones of the hands and feet are found in sarcoidosis. (45:383)

18. **A.** In beryllium disease, there is no ocular involvement. (45:124)

19. **A.** There is no lymph node involvement in beryllium disease. (45:125)

20. **E.** In some reported series, clubbing of the fingers is an early sign, appearing before shortness of breath. Pleuritic pain is common; many cases of asbestosis are found to have persistent dry rales. (21:352)

21. **E.** The diagnosis of benign pneumoconiosis is entirely dependent upon radiologic findings since, by definition, the patient is symptom-free. (61:102)

22. **B.** Clubbing of the fingers is usually evident in cases of silicosis and talc pneumoconiosis. Causes of benign pneumoconiosis include chromite and calcium. (62:140)

23. **D.** The Kveim test has been found to be uniformly negative in chronic beryllium disease and is valuable, therefore, in distinguishing it from "idiopathic" sarcoidosis. (37:666)

24. **E.** There is no specific therapy for asbestosis, diatomaceous earth pneumoconiosis, or silicosis. In cases of woolsorters' disease, even with therapy (penicillin or other appropriate antibiotics), death usually ensues within 24 hours.

25. **B.** In general, skin reactions are of little value in the diagnosis of extrinsic allergic bronchiolo-alveolitis (farmers' lung disease, bagassosis). This is true mainly because there are few suitable extracts available that do not cause nonspecific reactions. (41:366)

CHAPTER SEVEN

Environmental Toxicology

Directions: Each of the questions or incomplete statements below is followed by five suggested answers or completions. Select the BEST answer in each case.

1. In the industrial setting, which of the following is the most important route of entry of chemical agents into the body?

    A. ingestion
    B. skin contact
    C. inhalation
    D. parenteral
    E. ocular

2. A temporary blood disorder, methemoglobinemia, has occurred in infants following ingestion of well waters. This disorder is due to

    A. lead
    B. fluor
    C. iron
    D. chlorine
    E. nitrates

3. All of the following are simple asphyxiants except

    A. cyanides (alkali)
    B. argon
    C. neon
    D. helium
    E. carbon dioxide

4. Which of the following does *not* irritate the respiratory tract?

    A. ammonia
    B. carbon monoxide
    C. chlorine
    D. ozone
    E. phosgene

5. Which of the following has the least affinity for lipids and, in practice, is found to be the least narcotic under pressure?

    A. neon
    B. hydrogen
    C. nitrogen
    D. argon
    E. helium

6. All of the following phrases or statements referring to carbon monoxide poisoning are true *except*

    A. carbon monoxide is the oldest of industrial poisons
    B. there is profound tissue anoxia
    C. bradypnea is a symptom
    D. blisters and bullous lesions may occur
    E. peristent neurologic complications are common

7. The "cherry red" coloration of the skin, commonly believed to be characteristic of acute poisoning, is in fact rarely observed in

the living patient, though it is seen much more readily at autopsy. This statement corresponds with

A. carbon monoxide poisoning
B. hydrogen cyanide poisoning
C. phosgene poisoning
D. aniline poisoning
E. carbon dioxide poisoning

8. All of the following are convulsants *except*

A. strychnine
B. DDT
C. nicotine
D. phenol
E. chloroform

9. All of the following are neurotoxins producing peripheral neuropathy *except*

A. thallium (soluble compounds)
B. methylbromide
C. lindane
D. methyl butyl ketone
E. acrylamide

10. Which of the following is *not* a bone-seeking substance?

A. inorganic lead
B. radium
C. inorganic mercury
D. phosphorus
E. calcium

11. Inorganic lead poisoning is characterized by which of the following?

A. asthenia
B. weight loss
C. anorexia
D. pain in the joints
E. all of the above

12. Which of the following statements about the "lead line" is *incorrect*?

A. a bluish-black stippling that appears along the margin of the gums
B. these granules consist of black lead sulfide produced by contact of the absorbed lead with the hydrogen sulfide produced by the decay of proteinaceous material between the teeth
C. any heavy metal will combine with sulfur to form a black sulfide and thus confuse the diagnosis
D. it is a great help in establishing lead exposure
E. its presence means that lead is being absorbed at that time

13. Manganese poisoning is characterized by which of the following?

A. expressionless face
B. uncontrollable laughter
C. gait disturbances
D. micrographia
E. all of the above

14. Which of the following has been associated with a syndrome called "itai-itai"? It involves severe pains in the bones, waddling gait, aminoaciduria, glycosuria, decreased pancreatic function, pronounced osteomalacia, and numerous pathologic fractures.

A. organic mercury
B. inorganic lead
C. red phosphorus
D. cadmium
E. inorganic mercury

15. Which of the following statements about metal fume fever is *incorrect*?

A. a sudden chill and a rise in temperature follow inhalation
B. "Monday morning fever"
C. leukopenia occurs
D. resembles an infection by bacteria or a reaction to the injection of foreign proteins
E. caused only by freshly formed fumes from heated metal

16. Industrial phosphorus poisoning, known as "phossy jaw" is characterized by which of the following?

A. slow and insidious onset
B. usually begins with a toothache
C. the swollen jaw is extremely painful
D. suppuration is accompanied by a foul, fetid discharge
E. all of the above

17. Which of the following may be observed in workers suffering parathion poisoning?

    A. Cheyne-Stoke's respiration
    B. slurred speech
    C. ataxia
    D. excessive salivation
    E. all of the above

18. All of the following are cholinesterase inhibitors *except*

    A. DDT
    B. Malathion
    C. parathion
    D. Carbaryl
    E. methyl parathion

19. Which of the following is the first major step in the treatment of organophosphate intoxication?

    A. intravenous administration of atropine sulfate
    B. intravenous administration of 2-PAM (2-pyridine aldoxime)
    C. decontamination of skin and hair with alkaline soap and water
    D. evacuation of the stomach and gut if the poisoning has been by the oral route
    E. maintenance of patent airway

20. Occupational exposure to chlordecone (Kepone) in a pesticide manufacturing plant may produce an illness characterized by

    A. ocular flutter (opsoclonus)
    B. oligospermia
    C. muscle weakness
    D. generalized tremors
    E. all of the above

21. Which of the following statements about methanol (methyl alcohol) poisoning is correct?

    A. onset symptoms of occupational exposure to its vapors have included paresthesias, numbness, and pain in the hands and forearms
    B. the severity of the symptoms is believed to be proportional to the intensity of the acidosis
    C. visual disturbances are the most striking aspect of this intoxication
    D. survivors of severe poisoning may show mild dementia and a Parkinsonlike syndrome
    E. all of the above

22. Which of the following statements about green-tobacco illness is (are) correct?

    A. experienced by tobacco harvesters who handle uncured damp leaves in the field
    B. characterized by headache, nausea, severe vomiting, pallor, prostration
    C. the cause appears to be dermal absorption of nicotine from the wet tobacco leaves
    D. self-limited illness with recovery within 24 hours
    E. all of the above

23. Which of the following is *not* a sign of occupational exposure to fluorides?

    A. perforated nasal septum
    B. nystagmus
    C. hypertension
    D. mottled dental enamel
    E. hypotension

24. Which of the following might bind chlordecone (Kepone) and hasten its excretion?

    A. atropine
    B. calcium
    C. tannic acid
    D. cholestyramine
    E. pralidoxime (2-PAM)

25. It is important that medical care be obtained without delay in cases of

    A. masklike face caused by manganese poisoning
    B. hyperkeratosis caused by arsenic
    C. cholinesterase inhibition caused by parathion poisoning
    D. granuloma of the skin caused by beryllium
    E. metal fume fever caused by cadmium

26. Chelating agents now available are useless in the treatment of disease caused by

    A. lewisite
    B. inorganic lead
    C. mercury
    D. beryllium
    E. vanadium

Directions: Each group of questions below consists of five lettered headings followed by a list of numbered words or phrases. For each numbered word or phrase select the one heading that is most closely related to it.

Questions 27 through 31

    A. Phosgene (carbonyl chloride)
    B. Carbon monoxide
    C. Hydrogen cyanide
    D. Nitroglycerine, nitrobenzene, aniline
    E. Arsenic

27. blood highly viscous, thereby reducing blood flow and the rate of oxygen transport; erythrocytosis

28. displacement of oxygen from hemoglobin molecule

29. prevents tissue cells from utilizing oxygen carried to them

30. oxyhemoglobin is converted to methemoglobin

31. edema of the lungs; severe respiratory irritant

Questions 32 through 36

    A. Arsine
    B. Hydrogen sulphide
    C. Free silica
    D. Beryllium
    E. Altitude

32. acts directly upon the respiratory center of the brain, causing respiratory paralysis

33. hemolytic agent

34. alveolar capillary block

35. disturbance in the cardiorespiratory function resulting in a reduction of blood flow and oxygen transport to tissue cells; lung fibrosis

36. reduced oxygen pressure

Questions 37 through 41

    A. Osteosarcoma
    B. Osteonecrosis (phossy jaw)
    C. Osteosclerosis
    D. Osteomalacia
    E. Acro-osteolisis

37. cadmium

38. phosphorus

39. radium

40. fluorides

41. vinyl chloride

Questions 42 through 46

    A. Methyl bromide
    B. Tri-ortho-cresylphosphate (TOCP)
    C. Methyl mercury
    D. Methyl butyl ketone (MBK)
    E. Thalidomide

42. solvent: irritant of the eyes, peripheral neuropathy, dermatitis

43. fumigant: convulsions, peripheral neuropathy, pulmonary edema

44. sedative–hypnotic: peripheral neuropathy, embryopathy

45. plasticizer: peripheral neuropathy, gastrointestinal disturbances

46. minimata disease: paresthesias, ataxia, dysarthria

Questions 47 through 51

    A. Cyanosis
    B. Excessively pink color
    C. Bronze, blue-gray, brownish-black color
    D. Pallor
    E. Jaundice

47. arsine poisoning

48. aniline poisoning

49. carbon monoxide poisoning

50. hemochromatosis

51. lead poisoning

Questions 52 through 56

    A. Bitter almond odor
    B. Rotten eggs odor
    C. Garliclike odor
    D. Green tongue and metallic taste
    E. None of the above

52. hydrogen selenide poisoning

53. hydrogen sulfide poisoning

54. tellurium poisoning

55. cyanides (alkali) poisoning

56. vanadium pentoxide poisoning

Questions 57 through 61

    A. Silver
    B. Mercury
    C. Zirconium
    D. Arsenic
    E. Thallium

57. acrodynia

58. characteristic slate-gray discoloration of the skin; argyria

59. loss of hair from the scalp and the lateral two thirds of the eyebrows

60. cutaneous granulomas

61. keratotic lesions in palms and soles, and later may become widespread; these lesions may evolve into cutaneous carcinomas

Questions 62 through 66

    A. Strychnine poisoning
    B. Salicylate poisoning
    C. Chlorpromazine hydrochloride (Thorazine)
    D. Digitalis poisoning
    E. Warfarin

62. stiffness of neck and facial muscles; increased reflex excitability; tetanic convulsions with opisthotonos

63. causes hypoprothrombinemia and vascular injury, which results in hemorrhage; rodenticide

64. gastrointestinal disturbances, tinnitus and hearing loss, hyperpnea

65. gastrointestinal disturbances, photophobia, modified color perception, disturbance of cardiac rhythm

66. agranulocytosis, cholestatic jaundice, parkinsonism; antipsychotic agent

Questions 67 through 71

    A. Chrysotherapy
    B. Chromates
    C. Nitroglycerin (glyceryl trinitrate)
    D. Cadmium
    E. Mercurialism

67. pulmonary emphysema, anosmia, yellowing of dental necks, and marked proteinuria

68. aplastic anemia, leukopenia, dermatitis, stomatitis, jaundice

69. penetrating ulcers of the skin, perforation of nasal septum

70. stomatitis, neurologic disturbances, erethism, marked renal damage

71. the "powder" headache, hypotension, flushing, palpitations

Questions 72 through 76

    A. Sulfuric acid
    B. Chlorodiphenyl: 42% chlorine
    C. Phosgene
    D. Cyanide
    E. Perchloroethylene (tetrachloroethylene)

72. weakness, headache, confusion, nausea, vomiting, collapse; can cause rapid death due to metabolic asphyxiation

73. primary irritant effects on skin, eyes, and other mucous membranes and respiratory tract; corrosion of teeth

74. chloracne, liver damage

75. deadly war gas; pulmonary irritation, pulmonary edema

76. irritation of the respiratory tract and mucous membranes, narcosis, dermatitis, liver injury

Questions 77 through 81

    A. Lead (inorganic compounds)
    B. Formaldehyde
    C. Chromium salts
    D. Mercury
    E. Phosphorus (yellow)

Special tests:

77. increase in levels of delta-aminolevulinic acid (ALA) in blood and urine

78. patch test

79. routine x-ray films of jaws

80. serum creatinine, blood urea nitrogen, urine sediment, and other indices of kidney function

81. blood and urine levels of coproporphyrin III

Questions 82 through 86

    A. Methyl alcohol
    B. Carbon disulfide
    C. Quinone
    D. Vinyl chloride
    E. Toluene

Special tests:

82. the iodine-azide reaction with urine is useful in estimating exposure

83. liver function tests and liver biopsy should be performed

84. assay of formic acid in the urine; measurement of blood pH and plasma bicarbonate

85. analysis of urine for hippuric acid

86. inspection of cornea by slit-lamp illumination

Questions 87 through 91

    A. Arsenic
    B. Benzene
    C. Carbaryl
    D. Aldrin
    E. Warfarin

Special tests:

87. the blood concentration of dieldrin is helpful in determining the extent of absorption

88. detectable in hair for many months after it has disappeared from urine and feces

89. aspirated bone marrow may be acellular

90. level of depression of red blood cell cholinesterase

91. complete blood count, bleeding time or platelet count, prothrombin time on blood plasma, blood in urine and feces

Questions 92 through 96

Preplacement and annual physical examination with emphasis on

    A. The liver and kidneys
    B. The respiratory system
    C. The cardiovascular system
    D. Detecting a history of convulsive disorders
    E. Determination of pre-exposure red blood cell cholinesterase activity

If a worker is going to be exposed to

92. acrylonitrile

93. carbaryl

94. carbon tetrachloride

95. nitrogen dioxide

96. 2-aminopyridine

Questions 97 through 101

    A. Glucose-6-phosphate dehydrogenase (G6PD) deficiency tests
    B. capacity to metabolize tetraethylthiuram disulfide (TETD, disulfiram, Antabuse)
    C. Serum antitrypsin (SAT) deficiency tests
    D. Serum ceruloplasmin levels
    E. Latex agglutination test

Recommended for detecting

97. Wilson's disease

98. chronic obstructive pulmonary disease (COPD)

99. hypersusceptibility to hemolytic chemicals

100. hyperreactivity to carbon disulfide exposure

101. hypersensitivity to organic isocyanates

Questions 102 through 106

    A. Acetylcysteine (Mucomyst)
    B. Physostigmine salicylate (Antilirium)
    C. Pralidoxime chloride (Protopam chloride)
    D. Protamine sulfate
    E. Sodium thiosulfate, amyl nitrite, sodium nitrite

102. traditional cyanide antagonism

103. antidote for severe acetaminophen poisoning

104. cholinesterase reactivator used primarily as an adjunct to atropine in the treatment of poisoning caused by organophosphorate pesticides

105. anticholinesterase

106. binds and inactivates heparin

Questions 107 through 111

    A. Edetate calcium disodium (calcium disodium versenate)
    B. Deferoxamine (Desferal)
    C. Dimercaprol (BAL)
    D. Penicillamine (Cuprimine)
    E. Edetate disodium (Endrate, sodium versenate)

107. has high affinity for calcium and is used in severe hypercalcemia and digitalis-induced arrhythmias; it should not be used to treat heavy-metal poisoning

108. used primarily to treat lead poisoning (plumbism)

109. a potent and highly specific iron chelating agent

110. effective orally and is superior to other metal antagonists for chelating copper

111. antagonizes the toxic effects of arsenic, mercury, and gold; it is not useful in treating arsine poisoning

Directions: Each set of lettered headings below is followed by a list of numbered words or phrases. For each numbered word or phrase select

    A. if the item is associated with A only
    B. if the item is associated with B only
    C. if the item is associated with both A and B
    D. if the item is associated with neither A nor B

Questions 112 through 116

    A. Inorganic lead intoxication
    B. Tetraethyl lead intoxication
    C. Both
    D. Neither

112. severe gastrointestinal cramps and constipation

113. the lead line is not an early sign, nor is stippling usually found

114. the amount of lead in the brain and liver exceeds that in the bones

115. probably the only lead compound that can cause acute intoxication when absorbed through the skin

116. high intake of milk will prevent the intoxication

Directions: For each of the incomplete statements below, ONE or MORE of the completions given is correct. In each case select

- A. if only 1, 2, and 3 are correct
- B. if only 1 and 3 are correct
- C. if only 2 and 4 are correct
- D. if only 4 is correct
- E. if all are correct

117. Which of the following agent(s) may penetrate the skin, enter the blood, and act systemically?
    1. aniline
    2. parathion
    3. tetraethyl lead
    4. lead (inorganic compounds)

118. Which of the following is (are) well known to cause bone marrow damage?
    1. arsine
    2. toluene
    3. stibine
    4. benzene

119. Which of the following statements about arsine (arsenic trihydride) is (are) correct?
    1. the most powerful hemolytic poison encountered in industry
    2. causes headache, weakness, dyspnea
    3. causes abdominal pain, nausea, vomiting
    4. lowered or inversion of T waves on the electrocardiogram

120. Heinz bodies (small round erythrocyte inclusions) are commonly associated with methemoglobin and a history of exposure to
    1. organic nitrates
    2. inorganic nitrates
    3. aromatic nitro and amino compounds
    4. inorganic lead

121. The appearance of basophilic granules in the red blood cells (stippled cells) points to
    1. benzene
    2. carbon monoxide
    3. aniline
    4. inorganic lead

122. Tinnitus may be an effect of
    1. indomethacin (Indocin)
    2. quinidine
    3. aminoglycoside antibiotics
    4. quinine

123. Behavioral changes have been observed among workers exposed to
    1. carbon disulfide
    2. manganese
    3. tetraethyl lead
    4. mercury

124. Aseptic (avascular) necrosis of bone may be caused by
    1. chronic alcoholism
    2. pancreatitis
    3. sickle-cell anemia trait
    4. lead poisoning

125. Chronic exposure of humans to mercury causes
    1. stomatitis with excessive salivation
    2. psychic disturbances such as irritability
    3. fine tremor of the hands, lips, and tongue
    4. muscle weakness

126. Abdominal colic may be a sign of which of the following?
    1. thallium poisoning
    2. arsenic poisoning
    3. organophosphate poisoning
    4. inorganic lead poisoning

127. Which of the following statements about lead poisoning in children is (are) correct?
    1. most cases occur in low-income families
    2. most cases are due to tetraethyl lead
    3. it may be related to pica
    4. penicillamine is the drug of choice

128. Psychologic manifestations of manganese poisoning include
    1. impulsive acts
    2. euphoria

3. mental confusion
4. irritability

129. Metal fume fever may be caused by freshly formed oxides of

    1. zinc
    2. copper
    3. antimony
    4. magnesium

130. Atropinization is characterized by

    1. flushed skin
    2. dryness of mouth
    3. tachycardia
    4. mydriasis

131. Which of the following is (are) contraindicated in the treatment of cholinesterase-inhibiting insecticide poisoning?

    1. morphine
    2. aminophylline
    3. phenothiazines
    4. thiopental sodium

132. Which of the following is (are) excreted chiefly in bile and eliminated in the stools?

    1. carbon monoxide
    2. manganese
    3. nitrous dioxide
    4. chlordecone (Kepone)

133. Suggested in the treatment of methyl alcohol poisoning is (are)

    1. intravenous bicarbonate
    2. ethanol
    3. hemodialysis
    4. peritoneal dialysis

134. Reduced cystine content of fingernails is observed in

    1. rheumatoid arthritis
    2. cirrhosis of the liver
    3. some malignancies
    4. vanadium workers

135. In which of the following is the onset of symptoms vague and insidious?

    1. inorganic lead poisoning
    2. methyl butyl Ketone poisoning
    3. inorganic mercury poisoning
    4. "welders' flash"

136. Occupation may be an important factor in the development of

    1. anemia
    2. hypertension
    3. hypoprothrombinemia
    4. hypotension

137. Which of the following statements about the threshold limit values (TLVs) is (are) correct?

    1. time-weighted average values
    2. guidelines and are not intended as absolute boundaries between safe and dangerous concentrations
    3. no excursion above the TLV is permitted for substances that have a ceiling value
    4. the TLV does not take into account absorption of the substance through the skin, mucous membranes, or eyes

138. Biologic monitoring

    1. is an element of a program for control of industrial chemical exposure
    2. takes into account skin absorption of a chemical
    3. requires human beings as sample units
    4. is aimed at detecting individuals with impending or already evident adverse health effects

139. BAL (British anti-lewisite) is not recommended for treatment of

    1. tellurium poisoning
    2. selenium poisoning
    3. cadmium poisoning
    4. chromium poisoning

140. Metal antagonists have been tried unsuccessfully in the treatment of

    1. porphyria
    2. nephrocalcinosis
    3. sarcoidosis
    4. scleroderma

141. Trisodium calcium pentetate (DPTA) hastens the excretion of

    1. uranium
    2. polonium
    3. strontium
    4. lanthanum

Answers and Explanations
Environmental Toxicology

1. **C.** In the industrial setting, inhalation is the most important route of entry of chemical agents into the body. Next is contact with the skin. (45:4)

2. **E.** Nitrates, in concentrations greater than 10 mg/liter of nitrogen. The disease results from the conversion in the gastrointestinal tract of innocuous nitrates to nitrites, which then convert hemoglobin to methemoglobin (which cannot transport oxygen), resulting in suffocation. (37:988)

3. **A.** Cyanide is a chemical asphyxiant. Intoxication by a cyanide or a substance that yields cyanide ions demands prompt treatment of a highly specific nature. Argon, neon, helium, and carbon dioxide are simple asphyxiants. (45:50)

4. **B.** Carbon monoxide does not irritate the respiratory tract but is rapidly absorbed into the blood. Ammonia, chlorine, ozone, and phosgene are irritants of the respiratory tract. (61:97)

5. **E.** The amount of narcotic effect closely follows the Meyer-Overton hypothesis, which states that a parallel exists between the affinity of an aliphatic anesthetic for lipid and its narcotic potency. Helium has the least affinity for lipids and, in practice, is found to be the least narcotic under pressure. It is followed in increasing fat affinity (and narcotic effect) by neon, hydrogen, nitrogen, argon, krypton, and xenon, in that order. (63:365)

6. **C.** Tachypnea is observed in carbon monoxide poisoning. (45:151)

7. **A.** Because carboxyhemoglobin has a bright color, an occasional individual will exhibit the unusual combination of hypoxia together with a bright red color of the fingernails, mucous membranes, and skin. However, this cherry red color is usually seen only at autopsy. (45:151)

8. **E.** Chloroform is a central nervous system depressant that is toxic to the liver and kidneys. Strychnine, DDT, nicotine, and phenol are convulsants. (45:50)

9. **C.** Lindane is an insecticide and convulsant. In animals it is a carcinogen. Lindane has been suspected as a cause of aplastic anemia in a number of cases reported in various countries. (45:51)

10. **C.** Inorganic mercury has a cumulative effect and a tendency to deposit in certain organs, most notably the brain, liver, and kidneys. (45:320)

11. **E.** The onset of symptoms of lead poisoning is often abrupt; presenting complaints are often weakness, weight loss, lassitude, insomnia, pain in the joints, and hypotension. (45:308)

12. **E.** The presence of the "lead line" does not mean that lead is being absorbed at that time. In some cases there is no evidence of active lead absorption, as shown by blood and urine levels, so that the line reflects lead deposited at some earlier time. (21:74)

13. **E.** Among the symptoms of the established phase of the intoxication are speech disorders, expressionless face, spasmodic laughter, spasmodic weeping, hyperemotionalism, and clumsiness of movements. (43:241)

14. **D.** In Japan from 1939 until 1945, some 200 persons fell ill because of chronic cadmium poisoning. Drinking water and water for irrigation of rice fields was drawn from a polluted river. A syndrome called itai-itai disease developed. Half of the patients died. This is the most alarming indication of the danger inherent in chronic exposure to cadmium. (53:349)

15. **C.** The course of metal fume fever does not re-

semble that of an intoxication by metallic compound but, rather, an infection by bacteria or the injection of foreign proteins. The leukocytosis persists longer than the fever. Freshly formed oxide particles are finely divided and not yet agglomerated and so pass easily through the air passages. In a short time, however, the particles clump and will no longer pass with ease. This particle behavior is considered the reason that the metal fume fever is never caused except by freshly formed fumes from heated metal. (21:147)

16. **E.** "Phossy jaw" is caused by white phosphorus (occasionally referred to as yellow). Only a small proportion of the victims die. (21:116)

17. **E.** Early evidence of intoxication includes anorexia, nausea, sweating, substernal and epigastric tightness, heartburn, and belching. A greater degree of absorption produces vomiting, hyperperistalsis with cramps and diarrhea, increased salivation and lacrimation, profuse sweating, pallor, dyspnea, wheezing, and bradycardia. Miosis may be observed, but it is not a constant feature, since mydriasis has been occasionally noted. (45:399)

18. **A.** DDT is an organochlorine compound. Malathion, parathion and methyl parathion are organophosphorus compounds. Carbamates and insecticides such as Carbaryl do not require metabolic activation; they are direct inhibitors of cholinesterase. (21:289)

19. **E.** In severe cases of poisoning (coma, cyanosis), the recommended treatment is as follows: first, correction of hypoxia and cyanosis with oxygen and assisted ventilation; removal of secretions; maintenance of patent airway. (21:292)

20. **E.** Kepone poisoning is characterized by nervousness, generalized tremors, opsoclonus, muscle weakness, gait ataxia, incoordination, pleuritic and joint pains, and oligospermia. (21:296)

21. **E.** The symptoms are associated with metabolic acidosis. The physiological explanation of the vulnerability of the eye in methanol intoxication lies in the very high relative oxygen consumption of the retina and the impairment of retinal metabolism by formaldehyde, the normal metabolite of methanol, or, perhaps, by accumulation of formate in the blood. (21:204)

22. **E.** Occupational tobacco dermatitis also occurs and appears to be unrelated to nicotine absorption. (21:387)

23. **D.** Mottled dental enamel is not a sign of occupational exposure to fluorides but may suggest childhood exposure through ingestion. (45:42)

24. **D.** Cholestyramine, an anion-exchange resin that binds Kepone, has been used successfully to increase fecal excretion of Kepone by seven times. (45:36)

25. **C.** Treatment of organophosphate poisoning ranges from simple removal from exposure in very mild cases to the provision of very rigorous supportive and antidotal emergency measures in severe cases. (45:400)

26. **D.** The chelating agents that are used for the treatment of heavy metal poisoning are useless in beryllium disease. (21:32)

27. **E.** Exposure to arsenic under certain circumstances can produce erythrocytosis. (38:57)

28. **B.** Carbon monoxide reduces the oxygen content and oxygen-carrying capacity of blood and produces an unfavorable oxygen dissociation curve. (38:57)

29. **C.** Hydrogen cyanide can cause rapid death, owing to metabolic asphyxiation. (45:287)

30. **D.** Nitrobenzene and nitroglycerin may produce insidious, sometimes rapidly fatal cyanosis. In such cases the oxygen available to the tissue cells is reduced because oxyhemoglobin is converted to methemoglobin, which also has an unfavorable oxygen dissociation curve. (38:57)

31. **A.** The inhalation of primary irritants can produce edema of the lungs, thereby causing the individual to "drown" in his own fluids, which is analagous to drowning in the ocean. (38:57)

32. **B.** Hydrogen sulphide, at high concentrations, rapidly causes respiratory paralysis with consequent asphyxia. (45:294)

33. **A.** Arsine reduces oxygen uptake in the lungs, reduces the oxygen content and oxygen-carrying capacity of the blood, and reduces rates of oxygen transport because of cellular debris. (38:57)

34. **D.** Beryllium interferes with oxygen diffusion in the lungs. (38:57)

35. **C.** The lung fibrosis can be sufficiently extensive to distort seriously the architecture of the pulmonary bed. (38:57)

36. **E.** During the Olympic Games in Mexico City, several hundred nonfatal collapses occurred among the highly selected and optimally trained athletes due to reduced oxygen pressure. (25:84)

37. **D.** Cadmium poisoning is characterized by hypercalciuria, resulting from inhibition of proximal tubular reabsorption, leading to osteomalacia and painful fractures. (21:40)

38. **B.** "Phossy jaw" is an extensive necrosis, usually

of the mandible, which develops after a latent interval of anything up to five years after first exposure. (60:45)

39. **A.** Radium salts were first used in industry in the manufacture of luminous paint, which was then applied to watch and clock faces with brushes. The women employed in this work kept the point on their brushes by licking them, and in this way they swallowed considerable quantities of the radioactive paint. A high proportion of the women subsequently developed anemia and necrosis of the jaw, but, in addition, some also developed osteosarcoma. (60:187)

40. **C.** The daily absorption of 10–80 mg of fluoride over a period of years can lead to a condition known as crippling skeletal fluorosis, in which excessive calcification of bone results in stiffening of ligaments and fusion of joints. (5:141)

41. **E.** A feature of vinyl chloride monomer intoxication is the production of acro-osteolysis, which presents a triad comprising Raynaud's phenomenon, sclerodermatous skin changes, and lytic bone lesions. (60:91)

42. **D.** Methyl butyl ketone (MBK), a solvent, causes irritation of the eyes and nose and signs of peripheral neuropathy, including slow development of weakness and paresthesias; dermatitis. (45:333)

43. **A.** Methyl bromide is a neurotoxin and causes convulsions; very high concentrations cause peripheral neuropathy. (45:332)

44. **E.** Thalidomide causes a painful sensation in the feet and nocturnal muscle cramps. (53:598)

45. **B.** TOCP causes peripheral neuropathy, with flaccid paralysis of the distal muscles of the upper and lower extremities, followed in some cases by spastic paralysis. (45:495)

46. **C.** Signs and symptoms of methyl mercury intoxication include paresthesias, dysarthria, and emotional disturbances. (45:321)

47. **E.** Arsine is a hemolytic agent of extreme toxicity and with poor warning properties. Abdominal pain and hematuria are cardinal features of arsine poisoning and are frequently accompanied by jaundice. (45:111)

48. **A.** Aniline poisoning presents with signs of anoxia, including cyanosis of lips, nose, and earlobes. (45:104)

49. **B.** The carbon monoxide "cherry red" color is usually seen only at autopsy. (45:151)

50. **C.** The generalized hypermelanosis observed in hemochromatosis may be bronze, blue-gray, or brownish-black and may be accentuated in sun-exposed areas of skin. (16:612)

51. **D.** Facial pallor is usually a physical sign of lead poisoning. (45:308)

52. **C.** Hydrogen selenide produces a garlic odor of the breath. (45:293)

53. **B.** The odor of hydrogen sulfide poisoning is offensive and characterized as "rotten eggs." (45:294)

54. **C.** Tellurium causes garlic odor of the breath and malaise in humans. (45:457)

55. **A.** At high levels, cyanide acts so rapidly that its odor has no value as a forewarning. At lower levels, the odor may provide some forewarning, although many individuals are unable to recognize the scent of "bitter almonds." (45:189)

56. **D.** Vanadium pentoxide poisoning produces a green tongue, metallic taste, throat irritation, and cough. (45:504)

57. **B.** Acrodynia is a disorder seen in infants and children and presents with pain and pinkish hands and feet. Calomel intake has at times been associated with the disease. (16:1001)

58. **A.** The cutaneous effects produced by silver are local or generalized argyria. (16:1002)

59. **E.** Some 14 to 18 days after exposure, if the victim survives, the hair begins to loosen and fall from the scalp and the lateral two thirds of the eyebrows. (16:1003)

60. **C.** Granulomas result from an acquired allergic hypersensitivity to zirconium. (16:1005)

61. **D.** Cutaneous manifestations occur in acute and chronic arsenic intoxication. (16:997)

62. **A.** Strychnine is a potent convulsant. (45:449)

63. **E.** Signs and symptoms of warfarin poisoning include hematuria, back pain, spontaneous hematomas on arms and legs, epistaxis, bleeding of lips, punctate hemorrhages from mucous membranes, abdominal pain, vomiting, blood in feces, petechial rash, and abnormal hematologic indices. (45:508)

64. **B.** Gastrointestinal disturbances are the most common adverse reaction to salicylates: nausea, vomiting, and occult bleeding. The ototoxic effects (tinnitus, loss of hearing) are completely reversible. (2:94)

65. **D.** In a large percentage of patients, a disturbance of cardiac rhythm may be the first evidence of digitalis intoxication. Fatigue is the most common neurologic manifestation of toxicity. (2:502)

66. **C.** Thorazine has pronounced antiadrenergic and anticholinergic properties. (2:175)

67. **D.** Cadmium proteinuria and emphysema usually become clinically manifest years after initial exposure. (53:349)

68. **A.** Active adult and juvenile rheumatoid arthritis are the principal indications for administration of these agents. The usefulness of chrysotherapy is limited by toxicity. (2:105)

69. **B.** Chromate ulcers are round, punched-out holes that are painless and favor fingers and dorsum of hands. Perforation of nasal septum occurs in chromate poisoning. (45:173)

70. **E.** Chronic mercurialism, the form of intoxication most frequently caused by occupational exposure, is characterized by neurologic and psychic disturbances. (45:320)

71. **C.** The principal biologic properties of nitroglycerin are their ability to cause vasodilatation and to produce methemoglobinemia. The effects of absorption are observed in explosive workers, dynamite packagers, and workers handling cordite (a smokeless powder composed of nitroglycerin, gun cotton, mineral jelly, and acetone). (21:222)

72. **D.** Asphyxia and death can occur from high exposure levels, while weakness, headache, confusion, nausea, and vomiting result from lesser exposures. (45:188)

73. **A.** Two types of sulfuric acid injuries are encountered: (1) primary irritant effects on skin, eyes, and other mucous membranes and respiratory tract and (2) corrosion of teeth. (45:164)

74. **B.** Signs and symptoms of polychlorinated biphenyl (PCB) include eye and mucous membrane irritation, chloracne, signs of liver injury. (45:166)

75. **C.** Phosgene is a deadly war gas that causes severe respiratory irritation. (45:414)

76. **E.** Perchloroethylene causes central nervous system depression and liver damage; chronic exposure has caused peripheral neuropathy. (45:463)

77. **A.** The inhibition of delta-aminolevulinic acid dehydrase (ALA-D), an enzyme involved in porphyrin synthesis, leads to an increase in levels of delta-aminolevulinic acid (ALA) in blood and urine. (45:309)

78. **B.** Perform patch test with 2% formalin. (45:273)

79. **E.** In workers exposed to phosphorus (yellow) it is good dental practice to take routine x-ray films of the jaws, but experience indicates that necrosis can occur in the absence of any pathology visible on the roentgenogram. (45:418)

80. **D.** Mercury exposure: serum creatinine, blood urea nitrogen, urine sediment, and other indices of kidney function as necessary; assay of mercury in urine. (45:321)

81. **A.** In lead exposure, the blood and urine levels of coproporphyrin III and free erythrocyte protoporphyrins (FEP) are usually elevated. (45:309)

82. **B.** Approximately 70% of the carbon disulfide retained in the body is metabolized and excreted in urine as organic sulfates or other sulfur compounds. This analysis is not specific for carbon disulfide. (45:150)

83. **D.** Angiosarcoma of the liver is seldom recognized until fairly late in its course, within several months of death. Precursor physiologic alterations, which might be reversible, have not been identified. (45:506)

84. **A.** Methyl alcohol causes metabolic acidosis. (45:329)

85. **E.** Analysis of urine for hippuric acid, a metabolite of toluene, is useful in monitoring exposure to toluene. (45:482)

86. **C.** Chronic exposure to quinone causes brownish discoloration of the conjunctiva and cornea confined to the intrapalpebral fissure, small opacities of the cornea, and structural corneal changes that result in loss of visual acuity. (45:435)

87. **D.** The metabolite of aldrin is dieldrin, and the blood concentration of dieldrin is helpful in determining the extent of absorption of aldrin. (45:93)

88. **A.** A determination of arsenic in hair and nails may be useful, although its value has been questioned in industrial exposures because of the difficulty in removing all external contamination. (45:110)

89. **B.** The most significant toxic effect of benzene exposure is an insidious and often irreversible injury to the bone marrow. (45:118)

90. **C.** Carbaryl: The level of depression of red blood cell cholinesterase is a better indicator of a clinically significant reduction of cholinesterase activity in the nervous system. (45:145)

91. **E.** Warfarin: quick prothrombin time on blood plasma; blood in urine and feces; complete blood count, since secondary anemia (hypochromic, microcytic) may be marked; bleeding time or platelet count. (45:508)

92. **C.** Acrylonitrile is a metabolic asphyxiant with an action similar to that of cyanide. Preplacement and annual physical examination with emphasis on the cardiovascular system. (45:91)

93. **E.** Carbaryl is a short-acting anticholinesterase agent. Preplacement and annual physical examination with determination of preexposure red blood cell cholinesterase activity. (45:144)

94. **A.** Carbon tetrachloride causes central nervous system depression and severe damage to the liver and kidneys. Preplacement and annual physical examination with emphasis on the liver, the kidneys, and the skin; liver and renal function tests; urinalysis. (45:154)

95. **B.** Nitrogen dioxide is a respiratory irritant; it causes pulmonary edema. Preplacement and annual physical examination with emphasis on the respiratory system. (45:382)

96. **D.** 2-Aminopyridine is a convulsant. Preplacement screening questionnaire with emphasis on detecting a history of convulsive disorders. (45:100)

97. **D.** Although a blood test is available (serum-ceruloplasmin levels), abnormal copper is insufficiently sensitive to detect the more prevalent heterozygote. (55:565)

98. **C.** The "SAT" is of value in identifying those workers who are hereditarily prone to pulmonary disease when exposed to pulmonary irritants. (55:567)

99. **A.** In this case the fault lies in a deficiency in the red blood cell enzyme (G6PD) rather than in a deficiency of an essential biochemical substance. (55:567)

100. **B.** "Hypersusceptibles" to carbon disulfide are those with a reduced capacity to metabolize TETD. (55:568)

101. **E.** In the latex agglutination test, the isocyanate compounds, not the isocyanate antigens, are absorbed on latex particles. (55:569)

102. **E.** The use of the traditional cyanide antagonists is being reevaluated in light of recent investigations in Europe using cobalt edetate and in the United States using hydroxycobalamin. (2:1452)

103. **A.** Acetylcysteine, a mucolytic drug, is used as an antidote for severe acetaminophen poisoning (hepatotoxicity). (2:1452)

104. **C.** Pralidoxime is used primarily as an adjunct to atropine in the treatment of poisoning caused by pesticides that are organophosphate cholinesterase inhibitors. Atropine must be given first until its effects become apparent, and only then should pralidoxime be administered. (2:1455)

105. **B.** Physostigmine salicylate, a tertiary amine alkaloid, is classified as an anticholinesterase. It has been replaced in the treatment of myasthenia gravis by quaternary amines with similar anticholinesterase activity that do not significantly penetrate the central nervous system. (2:1453)

106. **D.** Protamine sulfate binds and inactivates heparin because of its strong electropositive charge. Paradoxically, it has anticoagulant action of its own and prolongs clotting time. (2:1456)

107. **E.** Endrate should not be used to treat heavy-metal poisoning. (2:1444)

108. **A.** EDTA is used primarily to treat plumbism. This agent is of questionable or unproven value in poisoning caused by cadmium, chromium, manganese, gold, and nickel, and is ineffective in poisoning caused by mercury or arsenic. (2:1445)

109. **B.** Desferal readily complexes with ferric iron to form ferrioxamine—a stable, water-soluble ferrous ion. (2:1447)

110. **D.** Penicillamine is an active degradation product of penicillin. It combines with copper, iron, mercury, lead, and arsenic to form soluble complexes that are readily excreted by the kidneys. It may be useful in treating cystinuria. (2:1449)

111. **C.** BAL antagonizes the toxic effects of arsenic, mercury, and gold. BAL should be used only in acute mercury poisoning. Although this drug also removes lead, EDTA or penicillamine is preferred. However, in severe lead poisoning in children, the combination of BAL and EDTA is preferred, since some studies suggest that this regimen hastens excretion of lead and reduces the incidence of brain damage. BAL is not beneficial in antimony or bismuth poisoning and should not be used in iron, cadmium, or selenium poisoning because the dimercaprol-metal complexes formed are more nephrotoxic than the metal alone. (2:1449)

112. **A.** In contrast with inorganic lead poisoning, there are no complaints of severe gastrointestinal cramps or constipation in organolead compounds poisoning. (21:80)

113. **B.** The lead line is not an early sign, nor is stippling usually found in tetraethyl lead intoxication. (21:80)

114. **B.** Contrary to the usual findings in death from inorganic lead poisoning, the amount of lead in the brain and liver exceeds that in the bones. (21:80)

115. **B.** Tetraethyl lead is probably the only compound that can cause acute plumbism when absorbed through the skin. (21:79)

116. **D.** There is still wide use of milk in lead-using industries to prevent poisoning, but students of the subject do not agree that one or two quarts of milk a day has a place in the medical control or treatment of toxic lead effect. (21:77)

117. **A.** Aniline, parathion, and tetraethyl lead may penetrate the skin. Inorganic compounds of lead penetrate the body by inhalation or ingestion. (45:308)

118. **D.** Benzene and toluene are excellent organic solvents. Benzene is well known to cause bone marrow damage. Toluene has no harmful effect on blood-forming tissue. Arsine and stibine are hemolytic agents. (21:2)

119. **E.** Arsine is the most powerful hemolytic poison encountered in industry. The initial symptoms of headache, malaise, weakness, dizziness, and dyspnea are followed by abdominal pain, nausea, and vomiting. A valuable observation confirming the direct toxic action of arsine on cardiac muscle has been provided by the reports of lowered or inversion of T waves on the electrocardiogram. (21:20)

120. **A.** Most nitrates produce Heinz bodies. Red cells containing Heinz bodies have relatively short life spans and appear to be preferentially sequestered by the spleen. Their persistence in the peripheral blood usually outlasts the associated methemoglobinemia. Inorganic lead causes basophilic stippling. (21:222)

121. **E.** In chronic intoxications such as those of benzene, carbon monoxide, and aniline, stippling of red cells may appear during the stage of marrow stimulation. It is a distinctive feature of plumbism that the number of stippled cells is vastly out of proportion to the degree of anemia. (21:75)

122. **E.** Indocin is a nonsteroidal anti-inflammatory compound with analgesic and antipyretic effects. Quinidine is useful in both supraventricular and ventricular tachyarrhythmias. The aminoglycoside antibiotics are so named because they are composed of amino sugars connected by glycosidic linkages. (2:98)

123. **E.** Behavioral changes may be caused by carbon disulfide, manganese, organic lead, mercury, carbon monoxide, and methyl chloride. (45:43)

124. **A.** Chronic alcoholism, pancreatitis, sickle-cell trait, and 15–20 other diseases can cause aseptic necrosis. (63:409)

125. **E.** With chronic mercury poisoning it is necessary to differentiate from other disease states with tremor, such as parkinsonism, cerebellar dysfunction, senility, hysteria, hyperthyroidism, drug intoxication and withdrawal, and Wilson's disease. (32:2)

126. **E.** A worker may respond with such severe pain and tenderness that the surgeon is induced to operate in the belief that he is dealing with an acute abdomen. (45:44)

127. **B.** Most cases of lead poisoning in children are associated with low socioeconomic status. It frequently results from ingestion of flakes of peeling lead-based paint from dilapidated dwellings. In severe lead poisoning in children, the combination of BAL and EDTA is preferred. (37:11)

128. **E.** The onset of symptoms is usually insidious: asthenia, anorexia, headaches, fatigue, muscular pains, mental irritability, sleep disturbances, sexual symptoms, and metallic taste. (43:241)

129. **E.** The great majority of cases of metal fume fever occur in brass foundries; the next most frequent source is the smelting of zinc. (21:147)

130. **E.** Failure of 1 to 2 mg of atropine administered parenterally to produce signs of atropinization (flushing, mydriasis, tachycardia, or dryness of mouth) indicates organophosphate poisoning. (45:400)

131. **A.** Morphine, aminophylline, and phenothiazines are contraindicated in the treatment of organophosphate poisoning. Anticonvulsants such as thiopental sodium may be necessary. (45:400)

132. **C.** Manganese and Kepone are excreted chiefly in bile and eliminated in the stools. (45:306)

133. **E.** Control of acidosis is essential in methanol poisoning and the use of intravenous bicarbonate

has frequently been life-saving. Ethanol may impair the metabolism of methyl alcohol. The availability of one or another form of dialysis and of rapid determinations of blood methanol levels and acid-base balance has dramatically improved the prognosis of methanol intoxication.

(21:204)

134. E. The cystine content of the fingernails of vanadium workers is reduced by levels of vanadium exposure that caused no detectable harm. It has been suggested that this finding might be used to monitor vanadium exposures or to aid in diagnosis. Similar reduction in cystine content of fingernails is present in cirrhosis of the liver, rheumatoid arthritis, and some malignancies.

(21:140)

135. E. The onset of symptoms is vague and insidious in exposure to a cumulative poison such as lead or mercury, or to a neurotoxic solvent such as MBK. Another condition characterized by a latent period of some hours is the painful eye irritation termed "welders' flash." Although resulting from exposure to the ultraviolet light emanating from an electric arc, rather than from a chemical exposure, this condition is encountered frequently among workers near a welding site, as well as among welders themselves. (45:41)

136. E. Anemia (inorganic lead); hypertension (diphenyl oxide); hypoprothrombinemia (warfarin); hypotension (nitroglycerin). (45:44)

137. E. The "Threshold Limit Values for Chemical Substances and Physical Agents in the Workroom Environment with Intended Changes" is prepared by the American Conference of Governmental Industrial Hygienists. Copies may be obtained, at a minimal cost, from that association. Address: P.O. Box 1937, Cincinnati, Ohio 45201.

(45:7)

138. A. Biologic monitoring is one element of a total environmental program for control of industrial chemical exposure that requires human beings as sample units and takes into account skin absorption of a chemical. Biologic monitoring should be distinguished from health screening; e.g., for anemia, bladder cancer, etc. (5:1)

139. E. Because there is no evidence that BAL is beneficial and some evidence to indicate increased toxicity, it is not recommended for treatment of tellurium poisoning. In selenium poisoning, BAL is known to increase kidney damage and decrease survival, and is therefore contraindicated. The use of BAL in cadmium poisoning is a matter of clinical controversy because of the reported renal toxicity of the cadmium-BAL complex. BAL has no effect in the treatment of chromium poisoning. (53:50)

140. E. Metal antagonists have been tried unsuccessfully in the treatment of porphyria, nephrocalcinosis, sarcoidosis, scleroderma, angina pectoris, calcified mitral stenosis, otosclerosis, and atherosclerosis. (2:1444)

141. D. DPTA hastens the excretion of lanthanum, yttrium, americium, scandium, and plutonium but does not increase the excretion of strontium, polonium, or uranium. (2:144)

CHAPTER EIGHT

Effects of the Physical Environment

Directions: Each of the questions or incomplete statements below is followed by five suggested answers or completions. Select the BEST answer in each case.

1. Bubbles appearing in the tissues of rapidly decompressed workers consist mainly of

   A. carbon monoxide
   B. nitrogen
   C. oxygen
   D. hydrogen
   E. helium

2. Which of the following is *not* related to decompression sickness?

   A. bends
   B. paralysis
   C. micrographia
   D. pruritus
   E. chokes

3. Caisson disease treatment consists of

   A. decompression and gradual recompression
   B. decompression and oxygen
   C. blood transfusion
   D. recompression and gradual decompression
   E. morphine

4. When the partial pressure of oxygen exceeds 2 atmospheres, which of the following may be observed?

   A. visual disturbances
   B. hallucinations
   C. vertigo
   D. epileptic-type fits
   E. all of the above

5. Air pressure in modern commercial airlines corresponds to altitudes above sea level of

   A. 2,000–4,000 feet
   B. 6,000–8,000 feet
   C. 10,000–12,000 feet
   D. 14,000–16,000 feet
   E. 18,000–20,000 feet

6. Which of the following statements is *incorrect*?

   A. noise-induced hearing loss is ameliorated by use of a hearing aid
   B. noise has been shown to cause alteration in the heart rate, blood pressure, and sweat rate
   C. greater energy expenditure is required to perform a task in noisy conditions than in the quiet environment
   D. the effects of sudden noise obviously disrupt work performance
   E. the main effects of noise occur at the upper levels of speech appreciation, around 4,000 Hz; with time and continued exposure, the loss extends to a range of 3,000 to 6,000 Hz.

7. Aging leads to a deterioration in sound appreciation called

   A. barotrauma

115

B. barotitis
C. Willis' paracusis
D. presbycusis
E. none of the above

8. In the United States, the permissible occupational exposure for 95 dB is

   A. eight hours daily
   B. four hours daily
   C. two hours daily
   D. one hour daily
   E. half hour daily

9. In the United States, no occupational exposure is permitted when the noise level exceeds

   A. 50 dB
   B. 65 dB
   C. 75 dB
   D. 90 dB
   E. 115 dB

10. Which of the following is the most effective and reliable way of controlling noise?

    A. ear defenders (dry cotton wool)
    B. reduction of propagation
    C. ear defenders
    D. control of exposure time
    E. noise reduction at source

11. Which of the following may be observed among workers exposed to segmental vibration?

    A. numbness and blanching of fingers
    B. loss of muscle control
    C. reduced sensitivity to heat, cold, and pain
    D. symptomless finger bone cysts
    E. all of the above

12. Which of the following may be observed in workers exposed to whole-body vibration?

    A. difficulty in maintaining a steady posture
    B. visual acuity severely impaired
    C. calcification of the intervertebral disks
    D. gastrointestinal tract changes in gastric secretions and peristaltic motility
    E. all of the above

13. Which of the following may be observed in persons exposed to microwave radiations?

    A. intellectual impairment
    B. insomnia
    C. irritability
    D. loss of libido
    E. all of the above

14. Human response is greatest to light in which of the following regions of the spectrum?

    A. yellow
    B. green
    C. orange
    D. deep red
    E. deep blue

15. The biologic half-life of a stable element is four days. Approximately what percentage will remain in the body 16 days after exposure?

    A. 75%
    B. 50%
    C. 25%
    D. 12.5%
    E. 6.25%

16. Which of the following can induce radioactivity?

    A. alpha radiation
    B. beta radiation
    C. gamma radiation
    D. x-radiation
    E. neutron radiation

17. Which of the following cells are more radiosensitive?

    A. muscle cells
    B. nerve cells
    C. bone cells
    D. lymphocytes
    E. granulocytes

Directions: Each group of questions below consists of five lettered headings followed by a list of numbered words or phrases. For each numbered word or phrase select the one heading that is most closely related to it.

Questions 18 through 22

   A. Heat cramps
   B. Trench foot (immersion foot)
   C. Heat stroke (sun stroke)
   D. Frostbite
   E. Heat exhaustion

18. occurs when there is actual freezing of tissues; edema, blisters, necrosis, gangrene

19. thought to be due to salt depletion: cool and pale skin, headache, dizziness, albuminuria

20. occurs in the presence of damp conditions combined with cold; swelling, pain, blisters, ulcers

21. the thermoregulatory mechanisms of the body begin to falter and the worker's temperature starts to rise; hot and dry skin

22. continued vasodilatation, with or without dehydration, will lower the effective cardiac output and lead to weakness, pallor, dizziness, fainting, and a profuse cold sweat

Questions 23 through 27

    A. Alpha particle
    B. Beta particle
    C. Neutron
    D. Proton
    E. Fission fragments

23. the nucleus of a helium atom

24. the nuclei of atoms produced when an unstable nucleus ruptures into two or more lighter nuclei

25. positive or negative electron

26. particle of positive charge emitted from nucleus or produced by recoil from neutron collisions

27. particle of neutral charge arising from the nucleus

Questions 28 through 32

Radionuclide
    A. Carbon 14 (as carbon dioxide)
    B. Mercury-197
    C. Iodine-123
    D. Phosphorus-32
    E. Gallium-68

Critical organ

28. bone

29. thyroid

30. liver

31. fat

32. kidney

Directions: Each set of lettered headings below is followed by a list of numbered words or phrases. For each numbered word or phrase select
    A. if the item is associated with A only
    B. if the item is associated with B only
    C. if the item is associated with both A and B
    D. if the item is associated with neither A nor B

Questions 33 through 37

    A. Infrared radiation
    B. Ultraviolet radiation
    C. Both
    D. Neither

33. nonionizing radiation

34. "glassblowers'" cataract

35. keratitis, inflammation of the cornea, conjunctivitis

36. has an important role in the prevention of rickets

37. is the most important part of the spectrum for the production of heat

Questions 38 through 42

    A. Alpha radiation
    B. Beta radiation
    C. Both
    D. Neither

38. complete shielding is afforded by a very thin solid material, such as paper

39. the whole of the energy is dissipated over a short distance

40. emitted mainly by radioisotopes of the heavier elements

41. detection may be difficult

42. interact mechanically and electrically with atoms in the matter they traverse

Questions 43 through 47

    A. X-rays

B. Gamma rays
C. Both
D. Neither

43. result from changes in the energy levels of the orbiting electron

44. extremely penetrating and theoretically have an infinite range

45. ionize gases and other materials through which they pass

46. electromagnetic radiation

47. normally generated by electrical devices

Directions: For each of the incomplete statements below, ONE or MORE of the completions given is correct. In each case select

A. if only 1, 2, and 3 are correct
B. if only 1 and 3 are correct
C. if only 2 and 4 are correct
D. if only 4 is correct
E. if all are correct

48. As the air pressure increases
    1. eardrums may burst
    2. alveoli in the lungs may be punctured
    3. severe sinus pain may result
    4. cavities in the teeth may cause pain

49. Which of the following is (are) observed in chronic mountain sickness (Monge's disease)?
    1. exaggerated level of polycythemia
    2. vacular occlusions in vital organs
    3. completely relieved by transporting the patient to sea level
    4. if untreated, results in death

50. Which of the following relates to Meniere's syndrome?
    1. hearing loss
    2. tinnitus
    3. vertigo
    4. always related to occupation

51. Which of the following statements about miners' nystagmus is (are) correct?
    1. poor lighting (semidarkness) is thought to be the cause
    2. only a minority of miners develop this condition
    3. symptoms include vertigo, headache, and sensitivity to bright light (photophobia)
    4. psychotherapy may assist some patients

52. Basic principles for control of external radiation (external-source radiation) include
    1. time must be minimized
    2. distance must be maximized
    3. shielding must be maximized
    4. minimize possible exposure by optimum choice of source

53. Which of the following statements about plutonium-239 is (are) correct?
    1. inhalation of contaminated air is the most important mode of exposure
    2. when taken into the systemic circulation, deposits predominantly in the skeleton and liver
    3. the trisodium salt of DTPA (diethylene-triamine-pentaacetic acid) is the drug of choice
    4. physical half-life is less than one year

54. The data on Japanese atomic bomb survivors show an increased incidence of
    1. thyroid cancer
    2. multiple myeloma
    3. breast cancer
    4. lung cancer

Answers and Explanations
Effects of the Physical Environment

1. **B.** The lowering of pressure causes a decrease in the relative solubility of nitrogen. If the rate of decompression is too fast, nitrogen comes out of solution too quickly and bubbles of gas form. (61:310)
2. **C.** Micrographia is not related to hypobaric states. Decompression sickness symptoms range from skin mottling and irritation to joint pains in the knees and shoulders. The affected limb is held in the semiflexed position; hence the name given to this condition—the bends. (61:367)
3. **D.** Treatment of the effects of decompression must start with the immediate recompression of the victim —preferably in a special chamber to a level at which the symptoms disappear. Slow, controlled decompression may then proceed, and tables are available for estimating the rate of decompression. (61:310)
4. **E.** Oxygen can become a toxic gas when its partial pressure exceeds 2 atmospheres. The toxic effects of oxygen are enhanced by exercise and carbon dioxide. (61:309)
5. **B.** At this altitude there is plenty of oxygen for the healthy passenger, but for the traveler with a cold this pressure may result in a bulging and painful eardrum. (46:339)
6. **A.** Unlike presbycusis, noise-induced hearing loss is not ameliorated by use of a hearing aid. Such devices, in fact, accentuate the frequency distortion. (61:311)
7. **D.** Aging leads to a deterioration in sound appreciation called presbycusis, which is greatest at the highest frequencies. (61:311)
8. **B.** The occupational safety and health act (OSHA) of the United States allows an increase of 5 dB for a halving of exposure duration. In 1969, the United States became the first country in the Western world to introduce industrial noise regulations, setting a limit of 90 dB. (61:174)
9. **E.** The occupational safety and health act (OSHA) of the United States allows a maximum of 115 dB. (61:174)
10. **E.** Minimization of noise at its source is the most effective and reliable way of controlling noise. (13:520)
11. **E.** The frequency range normally considered of importance for segmental-body effects is usually 8–1500 Hz. Segmental vibration primarily affects workers handling vibrating tools such as chain saws and pneumatic drills. (61:312)
12. **E.** The frequency range normally considered of importance for whole-body effects is 2–100 Hz. Whole-body vibration primarily affects divers, farmers, and construction workers. (61:312)
13. **E.** Microwave radiations are finding increasing employment as a means of rapidly cooking food. Mutagenic and teratogenic effects have also been reported. (61:306)
14. **A.** Response is greatest to light in the yellow-green region of the spectrum and least in the deep red and deep blue, so a lamp that produces red or blue light is less efficient in terms of visual performance. (61:196)
15. **E.** In twice the half-life the activity drops to one quarter; in three times the half-life, to one eighth; and so on. (61:283)
16. **E.** Neutron radiation is virtually the only ionizing radiation that can induce radioactivity. (61:286)
17. **D.** Blood-forming organs and reproductive tissues are most sensitive. Bone, muscle, and nerve tissue follow, in decreasing order of radiosensitivity. (51:33)
18. **D.** Frostbite occurs when there is actual freezing of tissues, with the cellular damage that follows such effects. Numbness and anesthesia, which precede frostbite, may mask the progression of the serious effect of the cold. (61:308)
19. **A.** Replacement of the water alone accentuates the salt loss, which is the biochemical precursor of the muscle cramps. (61:307)
20. **B.** Trench foot may be caused by long, continuous exposure to cold without freezing, combined with persistent dampness. (61:308)
21. **C.** The onset of this failure of temperature control may be abrupt, and collapse is then imminent. The body temperature may rise to over 40°C, with a resultant risk of permanent central nervous system damage and death. Cooling is urgently needed. (61:308)

22. **E.** In heat exhaustion the body's attempt to cool itself by dilatation of peripheral blood vessels is of limited effectiveness. Body concentrations of salt and water are depleted, and collapse of the circulation can occur. (61:307)
23. **A.** Definition of alpha particle. (19:121)
24. **E.** Definition of fission fragments. (19:121)
25. **B.** Definition of beta particle. (19:121)
26. **D.** Definition of proton. (19:121)
27. **C.** Definition of neutron. (19:121)
28. **D.** Critical organ of phosphorus. (60:32)
29. **C.** Critical organ of iodine. (60:123)
30. **E.** Critical organ of gallium. (60:68)
31. **A.** Critical organ of carbon. (60:14)
32. **B.** Critical organ of mercury. (60:197)
33. **C.** Electromagnetic radiation with a wavelength greater than 0.1 nanometer is regarded as nonionizing radiation. (61:257)
34. **A.** Infrared radiation can cause damage to the eye and is a cause of cataract development among glassblowers and others. (37:786)
35. **B.** Acute effects of ultraviolet radiation may be manifested as conjunctivitis, keratitis, and inflammation of the cornea. (37:779)
36. **B.** Vitamin D is produced by the action of ultraviolet radiation on 7-dehydrocholesterol or related steroidal compounds. (37:780)
37. **A.** The primary effect of infrared radiation is heat. (37:786)
38. **A.** Alpha radiation is of no importance as an external hazard. (61:286)
39. **A.** In alpha radiation, the whole of the energy is dissipated over a short distance. The maximal dissipation of energy means that alpha radiation from any source inside the human body represents a significant hazard. (61:286)
40. **A.** Alpha radiation is emitted mainly by radioisotopes of the heavier elements. Beta radiation is emitted mainly by radioisotopes of the intermediate and lighter elements. (61:284)
41. **A.** Alpha radiation, because of its minimal range, is difficult to detect and measure. (61:286)
42. **C.** They thereby progressively lose their energy and thus have finite ranges. (61:285)
43. **A.** X-rays result from changes in the energy levels of the orbiting electrons. Gamma rays are the result of transitions in the energy levels within the atomic nucleus. (21:314)
44. **C.** Gamma radiation and x-radiation, because they are uncharged, are not deflected by electrical forces and therefore travel considerable distances between successive interactions. They are thus extremely penetrating and, theoretically, have an infinite range; distance and/or shielding merely attenuate the radiation. (61:286)
45. **C.** X-rays and gamma rays ionize gases and other materials through which they pass. (21:314)
46. **C.** X-rays and gamma rays are electromagnetic in nature. (61:284)
47. **A.** X-radiation is the same as gamma radiation except that it is normally electrically generated. (61:285)
48. **E.** The body can withstand remarkable rises in pressure, provided that the air has ready access to all surfaces, including the lungs, sinuses, and middle ear. (61:309)
49. **E.** Monge's disease is a major high-altitude condition. Because of an exaggerated level of polycythemia, the circulating blood volume reaches high values and the plasma volume decreases. (25:99)
50. **A.** The triad of symptoms involving hearing loss, tinnitus, and vertigo is often called Meniere's syndrome. It is not related to occupation. The possibility should always be considered that noise-induced hearing loss can coexist with this or hearing loss due to other causes. (19:229)
51. **E.** Certain light-sensitive organs in the retina (the rods) are depleted. The condition is limited to underground miners, essentially coal miners; it is very rare in the United States. Defective vision has been postulated, but this is probably subjective rather than objective. (61:305)
52. **E.** Cumulative dose is a linear function of exposure time. Distance must be maximized. Shielding is largely a question of mass per unit area normal to the incident radiation. For external radiation, the three basic principles of control are time, distance, and shielding. (61:297)
53. **A.** The physical half-life of plutonium-239 is 24,400 years. Intact skin is a nearly complete barrier. (21:329)
54. **E.** The data on Japanese A-bomb survivors show an increased incidence of myelofibrosis, multiple myeloma, lung cancer, breast cancer, and particularly thyroid cancer. (48:310)